I0048650

PERSONAL & PROFESSIONAL DEVELOPMENT

FOR NURSING ASSOCIATES

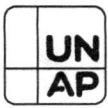

UN AP UNDERSTANDING NURSING ASSOCIATE PRACTICE

PERSONAL & PROFESSIONAL DEVELOPMENT
FOR NURSING ASSOCIATES

Karen Alred

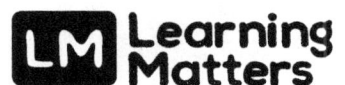

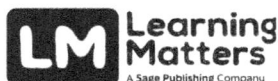

Learning Matters
A Sage Publishing Company

1 Oliver's Yard
55 City Road
London EC1Y 1SP

2455 Teller Road
Thousand Oaks
California 91320

10th Floor, Emaar Capital Tower 2
MG Road, Sikanderpur, Sector 26
Gurugram, Haryana – 122002
India

8 Marina View Suite 43-053
Asia Square Tower 1
Singapore 018960

© Karen Alred 2025

First published in 2025

Apart from any fair dealing for the purposes of research, private study, or criticism or review, as permitted under the Copyright, Designs and Patents Act, 1988, this publication may not be reproduced, stored or transmitted in any form, or by any means, without the prior permission in writing of the publisher, or in the case of reprographic reproduction, in accordance with the terms of licences issued by the Copyright Licensing Agency. Enquiries concerning reproduction outside those terms should be sent to the publisher.

Library of Congress Control Number: 2025939804

British Library Cataloguing in Publication Data

A catalogue record for this book is available from the British Library

Editor: Martha Cunneen
Development editor: Clare Weaver
Senior project editor: Chris Marke
Project management: TNQ Tech Pvt. Ltd.
Marketing manager: Ruslana Khatagova
Cover design: Wendy Scott
Typeset by: TNQ Tech Pvt. Ltd.

ISBN: 978-1-5296-9061-3
ISBN: 978-1-5296-9060-6 (pbk)

Contents

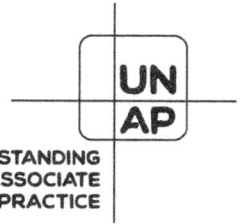

UN
AP

**UNDERSTANDING
NURSING ASSOCIATE
PRACTICE**

Supporting you through your nursing associate training & career

UNDERSTANDING NURSING ASSOCIATE PRACTICE is a series uniquely designed for trainee nursing associates.

Each book in the series is:
- Mapped to the NMC standards of proficiency for nursing associates
- Affordable
- Full of practical activities & case studies
- Focused on clearly explaining theory & its application to practice

Other books in the series include:

MEDICINE MANAGEMENT FOR NURSING ASSOCIATES

UNDERSTANDING PERSON-CENTRED CARE FOR NURSING ASSOCIATES

DEVELOPING ACADEMIC SKILLS FOR NURSING ASSOCIATES

Visit
uk.sagepub.com/UNAP
to see the full collection

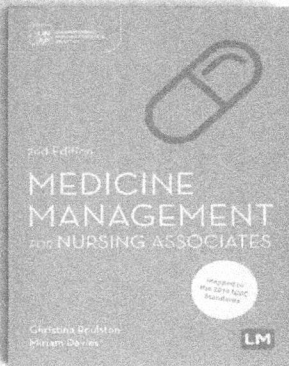

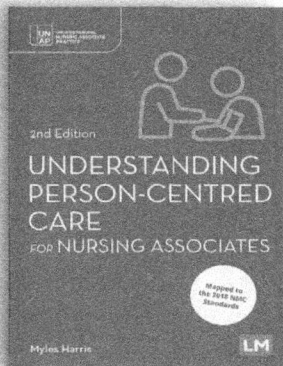

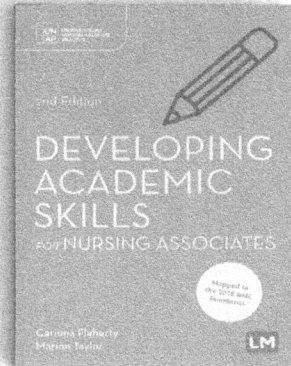

About the author

Karen Alred qualified as an Enrolled Nurse at Great Ormond Street Children's Hospital in the 1980s, completed the RN(A) conversion, and went on to become a Specialist Community Public Health Nurse in School Nursing, a registered NMC teacher and a Fellow of the Higher Education Academy. Past academic roles included Course lead for the Assistant Practitioner and Nursing Associate Higher Apprenticeships, and as a Lecturer on the FdSc Health Sciences (Nursing Associate Higher Apprenticeship). Karen previously supported the work of RCN Education Forum Steering Committee, is passionate about nurse education and supporting apprenticeships, using her own experiences of learning in higher education later in life to enable students maximise opportunities the Nursing Associate programme can offer.

Acknowledgements

This book would never have been possible without my inspirational mentor, Dr Sam Chenery-Morris, who enabled me to believe in myself early in my academic career. To Coralie Roll, my heartfelt thanks for your encouragement and support throughout our time working together.

I would like to dedicate this book to every Nursing Associate student I have worked with. Without your feedback on what worked and what didn't in class, I wouldn't have been able to refine the content of this book. I hope that one day, some of you will go on to become the future educators I believe many of you have the potential to be.

Introduction

Who is this book for?

This book is for anyone who wishes to apply and complete the nursing associate programme, particularly those new to higher education. It also offers guidance for newly qualified nursing associates, or others entering undergraduate study, to think about career progression.

About the book

Starting out in higher education can be daunting, particularly if you have been out of education for some time. This book is designed to support you navigate personal development, to enable your professional development. It starts by exploring your strengths, areas you may need to develop, opportunities that are available to you, and to help you identify how to overcome any barriers. I recommend you start by completing Chapters 1 and 2 as these are designed as building blocks for learning. This will build your confidence and create an ongoing approach to explore your potential and support your career through lifelong learning.

Book structure

Chapter 1: Knowing self and developing self-awareness This introductory chapter considers the importance of self-assessment, identification of existing study skills and how these link to professional development. The activities support this process to help you create an achievable action plan.

Chapter 2: Reflective practice Reflection and reflective practice are the cornerstone of nursing and delivering high-quality care to patients or service users. This chapter explores what is involved and why it is important to your own development, exploring some theory to think about different ways you can reflect in your learning and in your practice, while understanding your own potential for bias.

Chapter 3: Resilience for professional practice Working in a healthcare environment can be demanding physically, mentally and emotionally. There are many things that influence your resilience, and this chapter can support you to identify how this influences your professional practice. You will consider how you develop and maintain professional resilience, the link to potential leadership and how your organisation's resilience can impact on care provision.

Chapter 4: Role modelling and professional relationships Working in health and care requires you to work collaboratively within a multidisciplinary team. This chapter will help you think about how role models influence your practice and how you work effectively with others to enable high-quality care to be delivered. The impact of poor team relationships on quality is explored in context of the Francis Report and the Shape of Caring Review, where the role of the nursing associate was initially recognised as a potential opportunity to improve care in practice environments.

Chapter 5: Accountability in nursing associate practice The NMC standards and code of professional practice are explored to demonstrate the legal requirements of you as a potential registrant. The role of student supervision and assessment, responsibility and accountability as a student and registrant highlight the duty of candour. The scope of the nursing associate role and how this continues to evolve are explored in context of accountability and responsibility.

Chapter 6: Transitions and professional identity This chapter highlights the process of transitioning into learning, between year one and two, and into qualified practice and beyond. Using tools from Chapters 1 and 2, it highlights challenges you may face at times of transition to help you through these points in time.

Chapter 7: Employability skills This chapter helps you explore the skills you have acquired over the nursing associate programme, to recognise the difference between practical and theoretical knowledge, and how you use both within your practice. Understanding the extent of your knowledge and skills from novice to expert will help you consider how you apply for jobs or further study, drawing on Chapter 1's use of strengths and weaknesses and Chapter 2, reflection.

Chapter 8: Continuing professional development and NMC revalidation The focus of the chapter is on career progression, using a five-year plan to show how you can manage and control opportunities through the way you think about yourself, your knowledge and your skills. This links into NMC revalidation requirements and the concept of lifelong learning, along with the role and responsibilities of a registrant confirmer.

Requirements for the NMC Standards of Proficiency for Nursing Associates

The Nursing and Midwifery Council (NMC) has established standards of proficiency to be met by applicants to different parts of the register, and these are the standards it considers necessary for safe and effective practice. This book is structured so that it will help you to understand and meet the proficiencies required for entry to the NMC register as a nursing associate. The relevant proficiencies are presented at the start of each chapter so that you can clearly see which ones the chapter addresses. The proficiencies have been designed to be generic so that they apply to all fields of nursing and all care settings. This is because all nursing associates must be able to meet the needs of any person they encounter in their practice regardless of their stage of life or health challenges, whether these are mental, physical, cognitive or behavioural.

This book includes the latest standards for 2024 onwards, taken from the *Standards of Proficiency for Nursing Associates* (NMC, 2024a).

Learning features

Textbooks can be intimidating, and learning from reading text is not always easy. However, this series has been designed specifically to help the nursing associate learn from the books within it. By using a number of learning features throughout the books, they will help you to develop your understanding and ability to apply theory to practice, while remaining engaging and breaking the text up into manageable chunks. This book contains activities, case studies, theory summary boxes, further reading, useful websites and other materials to enable you to participate in your own learning. The book cannot provide all the answers – but instead provides a good outline of the most important information and helps you build a framework for your own learning.

Chapter 1 activities work together in sequence, with a case study to demonstrate how these can be completed. Many of these activities are repeated with different themes throughout the book. Reflection activities are supported with prompt questions, although once you have understood reflection models, it would be good to try and use one to structure your reflective activities. This will strengthen your use of reflection throughout your career. There are some student tips and reflections; these are from real students so you can see that you are not alone with your feelings and experiences.

Towards the end of the book, there is a glossary of key terms, which are highlighted in **bold** the first time they are used in the book. You may wish to consider creating your own glossary of key terms and their definitions to help you remember terminology. Remember to adjust your communication methods appropriately and to avoid professional jargon when having conversations with patients.

I hope you find this book useful in navigating your learning, both academically and in practice. Life has a nasty habit of throwing up the unexpected; hopefully, this will give you the tools and confidence to manage these so you can enjoy learning throughout your career.

Knowing self and developing self-awareness

NMC (2024A) *STANDARDS OF PROFICIENCY FOR NURSING ASSOCIATES*

This chapter will address the following platforms and proficiencies:

Platform 1: Being an accountable professional

1.5   Understand the demands of professional practice and demonstrate how to recognise signs of vulnerability in themselves or their colleagues and the action required to minimise risks to health.

1.13   Demonstrate the numeracy, literacy, digital and technological skills required to meet the needs of the people in their care to ensure safe and effective practice.

Platform 5: Improving safety and quality of care

5.9   Recognise uncertainty and demonstrate an awareness of strategies to develop resilience in themselves. Know how to seek support to help deal with uncertain situations.

Chapter aims

- Explore how developing study skills can impact the capacity to care and deliver quality of care.
- Understand the importance of self-assessment.
- Identify existing study skills to enable professional development.
- Identify relevant skills that enable personal and professional development.
- Consider how a personal development plan can identify the actions needed to develop study skills for independent, lifelong learning within care environments.

Introduction

This chapter will explore why we need to know about ourselves in order to then develop personally and professionally and the impact this has on our capacity to care and provide care – the themes of this chapter will be developed further later in this book, in Chapter 6. You will first explore your own existing skills and knowledge to recognise both your strengths and potential areas for development. This will then be analysed to create a strengths, weakness, opportunities and barriers (SWOB) analysis to further consider opportunities to achieve development, identify potential barriers and how these may be overcome (including systemic barriers experienced by people from diverse backgrounds and communities). You will consider how to look beyond your own perspectives of self to recognise how others perceive you, including positive cultural bias, and how this can enable or limit opportunities and progression. This will lead to the creation of a personal development plan using specific, measurable, achievable, realistic and time bound (SMART) targets (Doran, 1981).

Starting out on a programme of study

When you decide to undertake a programme of study, it can feel like an exciting time; however, it can also create feelings of uncertainty. This uncertainty might make you feel worried about how well you will do and possibly undermine your confidence. A way of managing this is to explore your experiences, knowledge and skills to see where you may need to think about getting help or putting plans in place to help you manage your studies and your worries. This can be done by looking at your past learning experiences to try and identify what you were good at and what you found difficult.

There are many challenges that people face through their early education, and it can be scary to think about that, especially if you did not have a positive learning experience at school or college. The nature of the nursing associate programme means that many people who decide to undertake the course have worked in health and care environments, often for a long time, but may not have a wide range of academic qualifications. Others may have had a change in career and have qualifications that are unrelated to healthcare. Whatever your past experience, you bring different knowledge and skills, and it is important to recognise that part of the learning you will undertake will include support of your academic learning needs. This book does not consider academic writing skills *Developing Academic Skills for Nursing Associates* is an excellent resource to support you with this. In this book, we are going to look at how you can explore your existing skills and address any areas that need developing but also to recognise your strengths so you can build confidence no matter what stage and level of study you are at. This links to building confidence in your own knowledge, skills and abilities and strengthening areas that require development as these impact on the quality of care you deliver to your patients or service users.

Study in higher education is different to school or college, and there are different teaching methods, particularly around independent study. The emphasis will be on understanding and learning how knowledge is created, rather than receiving information. You will be expected to manage your own study, goals and life and to seek advice and support to help you manage these. These are important skills to develop. As you progress as a nursing associate, you will need to be able to locate information to support your clinical decision making in practice to ensure safe, evidence-based care is delivered. It is also important to recognise there is a relationship between your development and interaction with your lecturers/tutors. There needs to be a balance of support so that you are not left to fend on your own to figure out how to overcome academic challenges for success (Gabriel, 2017). This is where knowledge of how higher education works can help you consider how to approach any challenges you experience in learning. Within practice, you will need to be able to ask for help or support at times, for example when you are faced with complex situations that are outside your competence. It takes courage to ask for help when you need it; practising this within your studies can help develop strategies, as well as the ability to recognise when and how you can achieve this. The first steps you take will help you recognise areas where you are confident or lack confidence with the different requirements for your studies. Exploring past learning will help you identify these and support meeting the NMC *Standards* 5.9 (NMC, 2024a).

Activity 1.1 Study skills identification

There are a number of activities to complete within this chapter. These need to be completed in order as they build on one another. Please complete Figure 1.1, the initial assessment of your competence for each skill. These will be revisited in depth later in the chapter once you have read more about each skill. Keep a copy of this as you will also use this in Chapter 8.

This is a personal activity; therefore, there is no outline answer at the end of the chapter. There is a case study that is used to outline some areas so you can see how these can be used.

The first step is to think about what study skills are needed for the Student Nursing Associate (SNA) programme and how confident you feel in meeting these.

Using a tool such as a study skills assessment scale (Figure 1.1) can help identify areas that you feel confident in and others where you may feel less confident and help you consider where you are now. There are skills identified as a starting point but others you may want to think about are personal qualities such as self-awareness and self-evaluation (explored further in Chapters 2 and 3),

Skill	0	1	2	3	4	5	6	7	8	9	10
Reading											
Time management											
IT skills											
Paragraph structure											
Sentence structure											
Punctuation											
Workload management											
Essay structure											
Referencing											
Finding information											

Figure 1.1 Study skills assessment scale

independence, determination, commitment, positive thinking, decision-making skills, critical thinking skills, memory and understanding information. By exploring your previous experience of study and thinking about some of the challenges you experienced, as well as successes you have had, you can contemplate what actions may help in developing these.

Remember that the range of skills will vary according to your past experiences and there is no right or wrong answer here. The important thing is to be honest, so if you have never heard of referencing you place an x in 0; conversely, if you have previously completed referencing and you have had feedback that you correctly completed this and you feel confident in doing it again, you could place an x for 9 or 10.

To help you, the skills from Figure 1.1 are discussed below to explore some ideas you may want to consider.

Reading

The sort of materials you read regularly and feel comfortable and confident in accessing will influence your approach to this aspect of studying. The higher up the scale you go, the stronger your reading skills may be. For example, 10/9 would be textbooks or professional journals, 9/8 may be more complex fiction books or broadsheet newspapers, 8/7 less complex books or tabloid newspapers, 6/5 websites or leaflets, 4/3 social media, 2/1 letters and cards, and 0 you do not read anything.

Some of the challenges for learners link to poor prior education experiences, unidentified specific learning needs, working in English as a second language, family dynamics and socio-economic situations. Technology has also created challenges as short pieces of information are easily accessible; if something is difficult to understand or not very interesting, the next piece of information is just a click away. The impact on reading for learning is that you may find it difficult to focus effectively for studying as the information is more complex and in longer texts. In practice, it is important to be able to read and understand sometimes quite complex information from patient records, guidelines and policies within your organisation. By extending your reading skills, you will strengthen your ability to apply these effectively to ensure competence within practice, to meet NMC *Standard* 1.13 (NMC, 2024a).

The benefits of engagement in reading help with comprehension, remembering and using information (Leighton Gamel, 2016). Accessing the library resource and reading generally will help you develop stronger reading skills. This can help with development of paragraph and sentence structure, use of punctuation and increase vocabulary, as reading requires you to understand patterns and meaning of words and sentences (Newton and Moore, 2010, p. 224). This will support refinement of your documentation in practice for NMC *Standards* 1.14 demonstrate the ability to keep complete, clear, accurate and timely records and 4.4 demonstrate the ability to effectively and responsibly access, input, and apply information and data using a range of methods including digital technologies (NMC, 2024a).

Student tip 1.1 Academic reading

While I have experimented with several study methods, including active reading, summarising, and taking notes, as well as using visual aids like mind maps or diagrams to arrange knowledge, I have found that taking notes enhances my comprehension and provides me with greater clarity regarding the specific topic or module.

Bukola, Year 1 student nursing associate

Time management

How well you manage your time will be a key point for managing your studies, work, family, friends, social life and any other commitments you have. You may feel you have strong time management at work but have a more relaxed approach at home. To complete this line in Figure 1.1, you need to consider where and when you will be studying alongside your other commitments. Start by evaluating how you currently use your time, before thinking about how you ideally want to use it – this can help you to organise your time more to feel in control and save space for the things you really want and need to complete. It is good practice to create a schedule, set priorities, and allocate time for different tasks. This should then help you prioritise tasks and allocate time efficiently.

When you have a lot of tasks to complete, with conflicting demands on your time, it can be easy to put things off for fear or worry about starting them. This, to a certain extent, is normal; however, academic procrastination has been shown to result in poorer patient care skills, potentially reducing your knowledge and awareness. Significant factors in academic procrastination include stress, social problems, not being committed, lack of guidance and support, and absence of time management. Another consideration is if you have a specific learning need – you may be more likely to procrastinate because of the impact this has on your executive functioning. How you manage these will be personal to you; however, skills analysis can help you consider what strategies you have that may help you manage this for effective study.

Understanding the theory

The phrase executive function refers to the skills required to plan ahead, achieve goals, have self-control, to be able to follow multiple-step directions even when interrupted, and stay focused on a task despite distractions. These have been shown to explain some of the relationship between procrastination and ADHD symptoms (Bodalski et al., 2023, p. 49).

Workload management

Although workload management is like time management, they do differ. It aims to ensure that tasks are completed efficiently and effectively, and involves creating to-do lists, setting deadlines, and asking others to do tasks. It can help you break things down into manageable tasks. Using to-do-lists, planners and timetabling different demands in your life will support managing your workload and being able to adapt this when you have a higher academic workload, for example when assessments are due. As a student nursing associate in practice, this will support and enhance your workload management skills to meet NMC *Standards* 4.5 demonstrate an ability to prioritise and manage their own workload (NMC, 2024a).

IT skills

Think about what experience you have working on a computer, either a laptop or desktop. You may need to create a Word document, a PowerPoint presentation, record audio or video files for your assessments. You will need to be able to navigate complex websites to locate online books and journal articles. Your education provider will also have a platform they use for sharing learning materials. You may need to attend online classrooms and interact with peers (other students) in discussion groups online. If you have only used a smartphone for emails, online shopping and finding out simple information, then you may need support with this.

The transferability of IT skills into practice is a key consideration for accessing and managing digital technologies as identified in both the *NHS Long Term* Plan (2019) – which highlights the role this plays in prevention and management of disease to prevent morbidity and mortality – and the NMC standards (2024a) which include the need to demonstrate numeracy, literacy, digital and technological skills; the ability to effectively and responsibly access, input, share and apply information and data; and to clearly record digital information and data; and provide clear verbal, digital or written information and instructions when sharing information; and delegating or handing over responsibility for care.

Finding information

This links into your IT skills. There will be specific sites, such as Google Scholar, that you use for finding information to help you with your understanding of theory and how this is used in practice, although evidence has shown that despite nursing students using information technology to locate information for academic studies, they lack the ability to critically evaluate the quality of the evidence for clinical decision making (Chipps et al., 2022). Therefore, you may want to think about how you use information from the internet as well as how you discern its quality and reliability.

Essay structure, paragraph structure, sentence structure and punctuation

How much writing you have done in the past will influence how confident you are with structuring information correctly. In Figure 1.1, the different parts of this point are separated out as you may feel confident in using punctuation and developing sentences but may be unsure about paragraph or essay structure. If you have English as an additional language, you may want to think about the challenges you experience as a separate item. You may have diagnosed or undiagnosed learning needs, such as neurodiverse needs, something that is common amongst learners and requires additional support, both in practice and the learning environment. Writing in higher education differs to other forms of writing you will have experienced, unless you already have another degree. This is where resources such as Flaherty and Taylor (2024) (see annotated reading at the end of the chapter) will enable you to develop these skills.

Referencing

Referencing is a specific skill required in higher education. You may have never even heard of this, or you may have used references in previous studies. Understanding the importance of referencing is the first step. It is linked to finding information and critical thinking, all important skills you will need to develop for academic study as well as within your practice. Your learning provider will recommend reference support, but a good resource is Cite Them

Right, although there are many, often similarly named tools, make sure you use the one you are directed to by your tutors to ensure you use the correct formatting.

Activity 1.2   Reflection

After reading through the descriptions, take 5 minutes to revisit and review your initial study skills assessment in Activity 1.1, study skills identification. Do you need to add in more points or details to your skills?

This is a personal activity; therefore, there is no outline answer at the end of the chapter.

Case study: Beatriz, part 1

Beatriz has just started the SNA foundation degree and been asked to complete the study skills assessment activity (see Figure 1.1) to explore what support is needed. As a 45-year-old of Portuguese origin, they have lived in the United Kingdom for 15 years with their spouse and children, English is the main language spoken at home. They have been out of education since finishing school in Portugal aged 15. Functional skills in English and Maths were completed 2 years ago to apply for the Nursing Associate programme. They work in a local hospital, where they were initially employed in linen services, before moving into a health care assistant role 5 years ago. Beatriz ranked their current confidence for each study skill as:

- Reading – 6
- Time management – 8
- Workload management – 8
- IT skills – 4
- Finding information – 4
- Essay structure – 3
- Paragraph structure – 2
- Sentence structure – 2
- Punctuation – 2
- Referencing – 0
- Written English – 4
- Spoken English – 9

Strengths and weaknesses

Student reflection 1:1

When I first started and we were asked to say what our strengths and weaknesses were and I thought, 'what, I'm not going to tell you what my weaknesses are' – who

(Continued)

(Continued)

wants to tell the tutor their weaknesses? But now, I use the learning support team at the university and realised that I need to understand what my strengths and weaknesses are so I can work out what I need to do. The team are the first important step as they know the guidelines on what you are expected to do.

Rose, 2nd Year student nursing associate

Having a clear picture of your skills and needs where academic study skills are concerned will enable you to develop these for improving both your reading and writing. You will find that those you work with will start to notice how you are improving your record keeping, managing your learning needs in practice and how this helps support your confidence over time.

Once you have completed the initial skills assessment (Figure 1.1), you can think about what your strengths and weaknesses are, what opportunities are available to you and the potential barriers to managing these. This is known as a SWOB analysis (Figure 1.2). Assessing your skills is beneficial in being able to judge your own performance rather than relying on others' opinion and feedback. Using your strengths can also enable you to overcome some of the weaknesses or barriers that you identify but most importantly, you can set your own priorities, which will help develop confidence in addressing those weaknesses and barriers. Through this process, you can increase your chance of successful skill acquisition and strengthen independence in your learning.

The first consideration is to be honest with yourself and remember that you can have something as a strength and a weakness at the same time. For example, you may have a strength, such as communication with peers in class, colleagues and service users in practice but you lack confidence in communicating with lecturers in university, or doctors and other health professionals such as physiotherapists, occupational therapists or speech and language therapists. You may also discover there is a barrier to continuing to achieve a strength, such as managing your academic workload or when staffing is low in clinical practice, and you need to prioritise patient needs over your own learning opportunities. Additionally, you might identify an opportunity to develop one of your weaknesses, such as academic writing skills and turn it

Areas to explore	Why this is a strength/weakness What and why are these opportunities and barriers
Strengths	
Weaknesses	
Opportunities	
Barriers	

Figure 1.2   SWOB analysis

into a strength for improving your documentation in practice. When you turn to completing your own SWOB analysis, include details as you want to analyse why you have identified each. This will help you think about how you can address the weakness or barrier.

Activity 1.3   SWOB analysis

Now you have your skills assessment; use this to complete Figure 1.2, SWOB analysis. Think about your strengths and weakness and identify opportunities and potential barriers to your learning. The box in column 2 is for completion of each element and why these are a strength or weakness, including what and why opportunities and barriers you have included. Keep a copy of your SWOB analysis as you will revisit this in chapter 4.

Case study Beatriz, Part 2 is used to outline some ideas so you can see how these can be developed.

The Johari Window

Once you have identified your own thoughts on your strengths and weaknesses, it can be helpful to get feedback from other people who know you. Other people will see different strengths and weaknesses that perhaps you do not see in yourself. One way of exploring this is to use a tool called the Johari Window, developed by Luft and Ingham, (1955) who explored how you interact with others and how others see you (Figure 1.3). This may initially feel a little uncomfortable, and you should prepare yourself to hear things about yourself that you may not necessarily think of as being you; however, by creating a space in your mind to explore this, it can be really helpful for you to think about yourself differently. The example of dyslexia will be used to explain each of the four areas.

1. Open Area is when you know things about yourself that you let others see. For example, you know you have dyslexia, and you share that information with other people openly.
2. Avoided or Hidden Area is when you know something about yourself, but you hide this from others. For example, you know you have dyslexia, but you do not want others to know that, so you do not tell anyone.
3. Blind Area is when others see things in you that you are not aware of. For example, your lecturer may see that you have dyslexia, but this is not something that has ever been identified and you are completely unaware that this may be something you have.
4. Area of Unknown Activity is sometimes referred to as the mystery self. Here you and others are not aware of certain behaviours or motives; however, we can assume they exist because eventually some of these things become known. For example, overcoming the challenges your dyslexia creates will later lead you into a role where you specialise in working with people who have dyslexia. These unknown behaviours and motives influence your behaviour and relationships.

	Known to self	Unknown to self
Known to others	Open area	Blind spot
Unknown to others	Hidden	Future or mystery self

Figure 1.3   The Johari Window

Activity 1.4   Reflection

Identify someone, either a trusted tutor or a fellow SNA on the course or within your practice environment to ask for feedback on your skills. You can then revisit the SWOB to enhance your skills evaluation and see whether there are additional strengths, weakness, opportunities or barriers to your learning that you can add to give a holistic picture.

This is a personal activity; therefore, there is no outline answer at the end of the chapter.

It is important to recognise that a change in one area will affect the other areas. It takes energy to hide, deny, or be blind to your behaviour which is involved in an interaction. Threat can decrease your awareness; however, mutual trust can increase your awareness. If awareness is forced, this is undesirable and would be ineffective in changing your actions, therefore, asking others for feedback can help you consider how others see you. This can be used to reflect on to help you grow as a learner, as well as work towards the requirements of the NMC *Standards* 1.5 (NMC, 2024a). You will explore reflection in much greater detail in Chapter 2.

Case study: Beatriz, part 2

Beatriz has completed the SWOB analysis openly considering some past challenges and how this may affect starting the nursing associate programme.

Strengths

I speak fluent English as I have lived in the United Kingdom for many years, and this is the first language of my spouse and children. I have good time management skills as I organise and manage my family's commitments, such as after school activities and work full time as well. My workload management skills have developed at work as we are often short of staff and I have extra tasks to manage. I prioritise and use lists to make sure I remember everything I need to do.

Weaknesses

I find writing in English quite difficult because the way English is structured is different. I sometimes need my spouse or children to help me with writing letters for school or other officials. I also find reading hard, even in Portuguese; therefore, reading in English is more challenging, even though I speak and understand English very well. This affects me being able to find information as well. I have never heard of referencing, which is making me worried. I do use the computer at work and I am confident in this as there are specific tasks I have learnt to do. I do not really use our computer at home. I use a smartphone for emails and shopping online.

Opportunities

My spouse and children all use the computer at home and write in English. They have said they will teach me to use this. When I completed my English functional skills, I was told about some help I could get from the council so I will see if this is still available.

My manager has told me the university has services to help students who have English as an additional language and for writing skills. My children have started getting me to read books to them in the evening so I can practice reading English. I am very slow but already getting better.

Barriers

I lacked confidence at school as I was not very clever, my teachers would get cross with me and sometimes I did not go because of this. I worry that the tutors will also get cross with me if I cannot understand information and that other students will not want to work with me because I am slow at reading.

Activity 1.5   Reflection

Within Beatriz's SWOB analysis, there are several areas where strengths may be used to support managing the demands of studying. The barriers identified are an important consideration.

Read Beatriz's case study and reflect on what areas you think Beatriz needs to develop and what actions may help with this.

See the outline answer at the end of the chapter.

Creating an action plan

Putting strategies in place to help you with study can make a significant difference to how well you do. By developing ways of working that are relevant to you, the way you think and work, and linking it to your strengths and the opportunities that are available to you will support you throughout your studies. These development areas can be expressed as personal goals on which to base an action plan (see Figure 1.4 for Beatriz's goals). Once you have a goal, you need to think about how you will achieve this and how you will know when you have achieved it. To motivate you in achieving a goal, it is useful to state this in the present tense and as a positive objective, as negatively worded goals can be less effective in providing motivation.

Activity 1.6   Identify goals

Now you have completed the SWOB analysis; list all the areas that you have identified for development. These will form goals for you to achieve.

This activity is personal to you; therefore, there is no outline answer at the end of the chapter. Examples of goals from the case study are outlined within the case study part 3.

Case study: Beatrız. part 3

Beatriz has used the SWOB analysis and the skills assessment to identify areas that need to be worked on to assist in development of academic skills (see Figure 1.4).

Development areas I need to cover in my action plan	Evidence/Feedback
To be able to access information from my tutors	Tutor feedback on learning
To develop my IT skills to find information in the university online library	Getting access to books and articles relevant to my learning.
To read and understand books and articles relevant to my first assignment	To be able to use the information I read in my assignment. Feedback from tutors.
To develop use of paragraphs, sentences and use punctuation correctly.	Feedback from tutors on a sample of my writing.
To use the learning from my first term to write my essay.	Write my first essay, submit on time. Read feed back from the marking.
To understand how to reference an essay	To reference my essay and get feedback from tutors and marking.

Figure 1.4   Example of identified goals

SMART goals

Using an action plan can help create clear goals which will then appear more achievable. It can provide you with a clear record of your priorities and provide you with a focus for your development. You should review your action plan regularly to keep it updated as your skills develop, as strengths, weaknesses, opportunities and barriers may change over time. You should be clear about what you want to achieve and how you will achieve them, therefore, they should be SMART (S = Specific, M = Measurable, A = Achievable, R = Realistic, T = Timebound) (Doran, 1981).

Specific

Specific goals are those that are clear and specific; they will help you as they are motivating.

Measurable

Measuring the outcomes from your goals is the only way you will know whether you have achieved it. Think about what will be different because of the actions you take, they may help you feel more in control of your life and give a sense of achievement.

Achievable

Achievability is a significant point. If your goals are too big, or would take a long time to achieve, then you will lose motivation. Think about how you can break goals down into smaller ones to help quick wins. This will help you gain confidence and further motivate you in moving onto the next level of the original, larger goal. Give yourself small rewards for achieving a goal, such as setting a goal of reading for 2 hours then reward yourself with a short break to do something you enjoy.

Realistic

All too often the goals set are larger, for example, you may initially identify passing my first assignment. To achieve that goal, you would have to access and understand all the learning from your tutors, understand how to develop a referenced essay, how to structure your paragraphs and information for it to make sense. To do that, you will need to be able to read appropriate books and journal articles to give you the information to develop academic discussions. To find books and articles you need to be able to find information in the library and through your university online library, which requires good IT skills. For this, you need to know what information you are looking for. To know what to look for, you need to access the learning materials provided by your tutors. Therefore, the goal of passing your first assignment can be broken down into several goals. Setting smaller, more realistic, achievable goals can help build on small success, which helps build your confidence as you build your skills. It can provide you with motivation and momentum as the goals are more easily achieved.

Timebound

When you have a specific time identified to achieve a goal, this can help focus your mind in identifying how you can achieve this. You need to be realistic about the time you have available – earlier in the chapter you looked at how to consider your workload and time management skills. Once you have some goals, you can start developing these into a full action plan (Figure 1.5). Each goal may require several actions, and each action will require its own evidence and timeframe.

You will need to think about how your goals link to wider goals, so when you achieve one, you are ready to set a new one that is a little more challenging. There are a few things that you need to think about in creating goals, such as identifying the implications of your goals, potential gains and losses in pursuing them. For example, Beatriz's first goal is to *Improve my IT skills so I can find information in the university online library and the learning from my tutors* (see Figure 1.5). The implication for Beatriz will be the time it takes to improve IT skills. This will require time on top of family life, working and studying, as they are likely to be prioritised over improving IT skills; however, knowing that taking time to do this will save time in the future can be a strong motivation. The decision will be whether a short-term loss of time now is more beneficial to gain more time for everything else in future.

This knowledge can help you identify strategies that allow you to recognise the benefits of actions and avoid negative outcomes. One strategy for building on this is to keep a reflective journal. You will be looking at **reflection** in Chapter 2, but it can be useful to reflect on your learning as well. If you note down your successes, you will be able to replicate these in future and be able to look back and see how far you have come.

Student tip 1.2 Self-reflection

I wouldn't normally self-reflect, but after taking the Personal and Professional Development module in year 1, I started to be more deliberate and do more self-reflection, both at work and when evaluating my academic performance and identifying areas where I need to improve. I set reasonable goals and track my progress to help me achieve these goals.

I make every effort to maintain organisation, but I also attempt to be flexible enough to change when necessary to avoid becoming overwhelmed.

Bukola, 2nd Year student nursing associate

Activity 1.7   Personal development plan

Referring back to Activities 1.1, 1.2 and 1.6, identify what you want and need to be able to achieve for successful study – you may also want to use the structure Beatriz uses in Figure 1.5 as a template for your Personal Development Plan. Consider how you can break each goal down to apply SMART principles to these. Pay particular attention to being realistic and achievable within the time frame you identify.

This is a personal activity; therefore, there is no outline answer at the end of the chapter.

Examples of Beatriz's Personal Development Plan are outlined within the case study part 4.

Achieving your goals

Sometimes it can be hard to accept that you might achieve your goals, and some of you may even have patterns of behaviour that sabotage your plans. It can be hard to accept you might succeed where in the past you have struggled with learning. You may start to blame yourself for past failures and think that you needed to try harder. Alternatively, you may feel that if you fail now, at the start, it gets the failure out of the way, as waiting to see if you have succeeded is too difficult. You may have a diagnosed or undiagnosed Specific Learning Difference (SpLD) which you may not wish to disclose. Knowing some of the behaviours that show this can help you recognise whether this is something you do. Some examples of this include not turning up to lectures, leaving academic work until the last minute and missing deadlines, filling up your time doing everything except studying (procrastination) and not using the university resources there to help you. If you know this is something you may experience, think about what things you are most likely to do to sabotage your studies, identify which experiences are most likely to trigger this and ask yourself whether you would recognise and admit that you are doing this. Now consider whether there is anybody you trust to share this with; you are likely to have a personal advisor, but your university or college will also have student support services who will be experienced in supporting students through these challenges. The secret is to tell someone before you start then you can work together to identify ways you can help yourself. If you have SpLD, there are lots of resources and support that will be available to you. It is important that you approach your education provider to get this assessed so that support can be put in place. This is called *reasonable adjustments* and are to ensure you have fair and equal access to learning, teaching and assessment. You could include this in your personal development plan.

Case study: Beatriz, part 4

Beatriz has completed a personal development plan, some of which is shown here to demonstrate how you can identify and break down goals and the actions needed to achieve those goals.

Goal/Target	Action	Evidence	Target date
Improve my IT skills so I can find information in the university online library and the learning from my tutors	Access classes on developing IT skills available through the county council	Enrolment on the course	2 week's time
	Practice accessing the university learning online	The system at the university lets me know where I am in the site and what I have accessed	2 week's time
	Access help from the university student learning services	Email contact with the service	1 week's time
To read and understand books and articles relevant to my first assignment	Go to the university library and find books on the reading list	Books on the reading list booked out onto my library card	1 week's time
	Read books and take notes from these	Notes to use for review when preparing my assignment	3 week's time
	Meet personal advisor to check I have understood information correctly	Meeting booked and feedback received	5 week's time
To develop use of paragraphs, sentences and use punctuation correctly.	Read more books and articles	Books and articles taken out of the library/accessed online	4 week's time
	Write a sample piece for my tutor to feedback	Feedback from my tutor	4 week's time
	Access the university help for English as an additional language	Book an appointment with the university support team	2 week's time

Figure 1.5 Personal development plan

Activity 1.8   Reflection

Reflect on this personal development plan (Figure 1.5) to consider whether Beatriz has identified SMART goals and what shows this.

Revisit your own personal development plan and reflect on whether this can be broken down into smaller goals and shorter, more achievable actions.

Have you identified a specific time frame to achieve these or do you need to revisit any of them?

See outline answer for Beatriz's SMART goals at the end of the chapter.

It is important to remember that embarking on a new adventure is in addition to everything else you already have going on in your life. Life can present many challenges, and it is important to recognise these alongside the additional pressure of studying. You never know what is around the corner and completing a 2-year programme of study may result in unexpected life events both big and small. Awareness of situations, such as major life events, as well as the daily hassles we experience, such as the school run or the car not starting, need to be considered and, where possible, planned for. There are also long-lasting structural and cultural situations such as poverty, unemployment and marginalisation which create strain for people. If you can consider all this and plan how they may be managed, then you are more likely to be able to navigate the experience as you will not face having to work out what to do at the time. This relates to the *Standards of Proficiency for Nursing Associates* (NMC, 2024a) to recognise uncertainty and demonstrate an awareness of strategies to develop **resilience** in themselves. Knowing how to seek support to help deal with uncertain situations will be explored in Chapter 3 on resilience.

Once you have identified goals and actions to enable management of your studies, you have taken the first steps to managing these effectively. This will help you work towards the requirement to develop adequate literacy, numeracy and digital skills necessary for safe practice, as well as recognise how you can manage your own needs and how these can be supported (NMC, 2024a). It is important to remember the purpose of completing your studies is not just for your personal and professional growth. Although this is a strong reason for studying, the reason why services want and need well-educated and qualified staff is to provide safe and effective patient care. This was the result of the Francis Report (Mid Staffordshire NHS Foundation Trust Public Inquiry, 2013), that led to the Shape of Caring Review headed by Lord Willis (Health Education England, 2015). These reports highlighted the gap between the role of the registered nurse and the health care assistant, which left patients at risk of not having their needs met. By committing to your studies, you are also committing to developing your practice to improve patient care and supporting organisations that provide care in both health and care services to meet the duty of care required of them. This brings with it a level of responsibility which you will explore in Chapter 5.

Chapter summary

This chapter has explored your own study experiences to highlight existing skills and areas where you need to develop. The activities have considered different skills, some of which you may have as both a strength and a weakness. Using the opportunities available to you, and recognising potential barriers, has helped to consider goals you want to achieve. Creating a personal development plan and applying SMART principles will help you create small, achievable goals.

The process of developing an ability to look at yourself and seek feedback from others are the first steps you will take towards independence in your learning, as well as starting to think about yourself and your learning needs critically. Keep an open mind to learning, feedback and experiences as all, including negative experiences, create learning opportunities. You will be likely to learn more from your mistakes than your successes, so embrace these. In completing these activities, you may identify something that may indicate that you have an underlying SpLD. This is your career opportunity, and you need to make the most of this. If you decide not to seek support, then see if you can find self-help information such as Malpas (2017), identified in the annotated reading at the end of this chapter.

Activities: Brief outline answers

Activity 1.5 Reflection (page 11)

Beatriz will need to get help with IT skills, reading and writing in English. They could access support through the education provider, their employer or the local council. Using their good organisational skills will help them make the time to complete this. Referencing skills is something they will learn as they go through the learning but they could also go to student support services for extra help.

Activity 1.8 Reflection (page 16)

Beatriz has some good goals that will help address some of the challenges faced. These have been broken down into smaller actions and clear evidence on how they will know when this is achieved. They have given short timeframes to make sure they can manage everything. Beatriz stated a strength was organisation skills and prioritisation so they have created different goals with longer timeframes as well.

Annotated further reading

Flaherty, C. and Taylor, M. (Eds) (2024) *Developing Academic Skills for Nursing Associates, 2nd edition*. London: Learning Matters.

This book will help you in considering some of the academic skills that you will need. It also thinks about your experience of entering higher education and developing academic skills.

Leighton Gamel, A. (2016) *Learning Vital Reading Strategies: A Workbook for Students*. Lanham, Maryland: Rowman & Littlefield Publishers.

This workbook has been designed specifically to assist students in developing their reading skills. It recognises that there are a number of experiences through early life that impact on the ability to read effectively, with the aim of enabling you to access texts and engage with them as this is an essential skill for academic learning.

Malpas, M.D. (2017) *Self-Fulfilment with Dyslexia: A Blueprint for Success.* [N.p.]: Jessica Kingsley Publishers.

This book will help anyone with SpLD explore their own potential through focusing on the strengths of the individual rather than trying to address specific areas such as reading or writing. It highlights key themes that are needed for success; if you have, or suspect you have an SpLD, you may want to consider linking your personal development plan goals to these.

Chapter 2

Reflective practice

NMC (2024A) STANDARDS OF PROFICIENCY FOR NURSING ASSOCIATES

This chapter will address the following platforms and proficiencies.

Platform 1: Being an accountable professional

1.15 Take responsibility for continuous self-reflection, seeking and responding to support and feedback to develop professional knowledge and skills.

Platform 4: Working in teams

4.7 Support, supervise and act as a **role model** to nursing associate students, healthcare support workers and those new to care roles, review the quality of the care they provide, promoting reflection and providing constructive feedback.

4.8 Contribute to team reflection activities, to promote improvements in practice and services.

Annex A 5.4 encouragement to colleagues that helps them to reflect on their practice.

Chapter aims

- Explore what reflection is and what it involves.
- Identify key reasons why we reflect and why this is important to your practice and learning.
- Understand how we reflect through examining theory.
- Discuss the range of reflective approaches available to practitioners.
- Explore Gibbs' model of reflection.
- Explore Rolfe's model of reflection.
- Identify the role of unconscious bias on reflective activities.

Introduction

Chapter 2 will build on Chapter 1 through exploring reflection, what it is and the different types and ways of reflecting. It will start by considering informal reflection of everyday life to demystify the process and to contextualise how personal experiences impact on professional beliefs and **values**. Now that you have identified your study skills and created a personal development plan, it is important to consider how reflection can enable you to strengthen your analysis of your knowledge and skills. This is also a required and essential element of professional practice as a nursing associate. This chapter will introduce you to reflection – how we reflect, when we reflect and how you can use reflection both formally and informally, individually and as part of a group. This will be completed through introducing three reflective models and linking through to a range of others. You will explore the strengths and limitations of each model and see how these can be applied to both practice and your academic development. It can feel a little challenging when you first start reflecting formally; it takes practice and commitment to use the tools effectively. Therefore, the activities and case studies in this chapter will aid you in developing both the knowledge and skills needed for effective reflective practice. This underpins professional practice, as required by the NMC for **lifelong learning**; however, challenges with reflection can undermine how you think about using reflection. This will lead to identifying the role of reflexivity and how this differs from reflection.

Reflection: What it is and why is it important?

When you think about reflection in its broadest sense, you can think of many different points of view.

Activity 2.1   Reflection

Take a few minutes to think about what the term 'reflection' means and what you associate this with. This will vary depending on where you are in your learning journey; if you are a registered practitioner, you may be contemplating revalidation, whereas a new student nursing associate may not yet have come across this.

Does this have different meanings for you in different places and at different times?

Why do you reflect?

When do you consciously reflect?

How do you consciously reflect?

The outline answer at the end of the chapter shows some examples but is very individual, so yours will be different.

One of the main reasons we reflect is to help us learn, mainly from experiences and often after making a mistake, or to avoid this when we can see there is a risk of a mistake being made. There are several theories involved in understanding how we learn. Understanding the process of learning will help you think about how you learn through reflection.

Bloom's taxonomy of learning

One of the main theories is called the taxonomy of learning (Bloom, 1956). Sometimes the term 'hierarchy' is used. Bloom identified that not all learning is the same – there are different levels to learning, and he named six levels (remembering, understanding, applying, analysing, evaluating and creating) (see Figure 2.1).

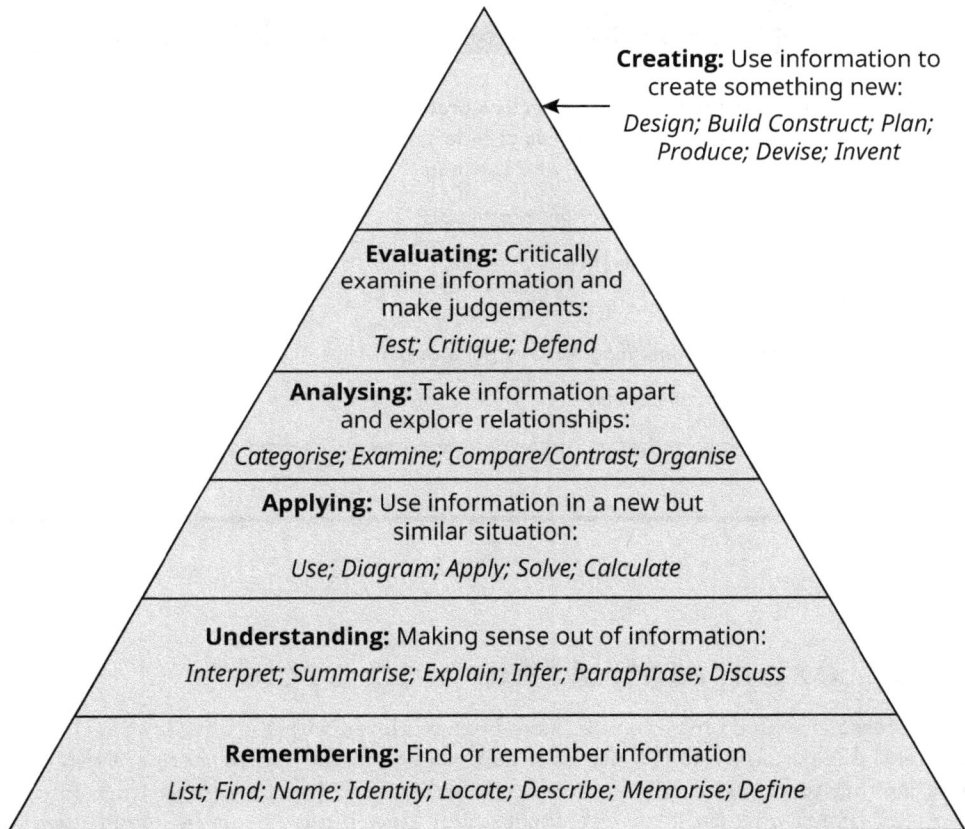

Creating: Use information to create something new:

Design; Build Construct; Plan; Produce; Devise; Invent

Evaluating: Critically examine information and make judgements:

Test; Critique; Defend

Analysing: Take information apart and explore relationships:

Categorise; Examine; Compare/Contrast; Organise

Applying: Use information in a new but similar situation:

Use; Diagram; Apply; Solve; Calculate

Understanding: Making sense out of information:

Interpret; Summarise; Explain; Infer; Paraphrase; Discuss

Remembering: Find or remember information

List; Find; Name; Identity; Locate; Describe; Memorise; Define

Figure 2.1   Bloom's hierarchy of learning

Level 1 (the bottom layer of the triangle) is remembering – memorising information; for example, Bloom's taxonomy of learning has six stages, so you see this image and you process this information as you can see six different levels, so you understand it. Next you need to think about application, so you may decide to write about this in your assignment. The top three levels (analysing, evaluating and creating) are then higher order thinking, so you now need to take your new knowledge and do something with it!

You may think about this to identify the relationship between Bloom's taxonomy and your own learning to then critically think what you may need to evaluate whether you have 'got it'. For example, you would have used this in your SWOB analysis task in Chapter 1. Eventually, you use it to create something new; for example, you may decide to produce a new learning plan as a result of your analysis and evaluation.

Initially, you need to identify which level you want to get to – like all goals it is worth breaking down into smaller goals, so you proceed through the different stages to master these as you go. You may also have different levels at different times, so for your Personal Development Plan you may have found this analysis easier than you did writing your assessment.

Activity 2.2 Reflection in practice

Healthcare requires practitioners to reflect as a process for learning. Consider these questions to explore your own personal experiences of reflection and consider whether there may be a different approach that may enhance your learning.

What are your experiences of reflection in practice?

Have you reflected with other people?

Do you reflect regularly on your actions?

Do you only reflect when something has not gone to plan?

Do you write down your reflections?

This activity is a personal reflection, so the outline answer at the end of the chapter provides guidance only.

Kolb's experiential learning cycle

The processes involved in reflection have been explored with Kolb (1984) developing an experiential learning cycle (Figure 2.2). You can see in the centre there are two continuums moving top to bottom from a concrete experience (feeling) to abstract conceptualism (thinking) and right to left observation (watching) to active experimentation (doing). Kolb recognised these as a cyclical process and advocated that you continuously gain knowledge through experience by testing new knowledge within those experiences. Kolb (2015) has continued to develop this process to recognise that within the concrete experience, you grasp understanding through worrying about your learning, which links to your feelings. As identified in Chapter 1, you may have negative experiences in previous learning experiences, which creates this worry. As you work through reflective observation, thinking about what you have observed and what it means, you intentionally transform to reach abstract conceptualisation, where you are able to make sense and grasp through understanding. This then allows you to start active experimentation by testing out your new knowledge, putting it into action, and extending your transformation. Over time, you accommodate this new knowledge and experience to return to the concrete experience, with new insight that highlights additional areas you may need to develop.

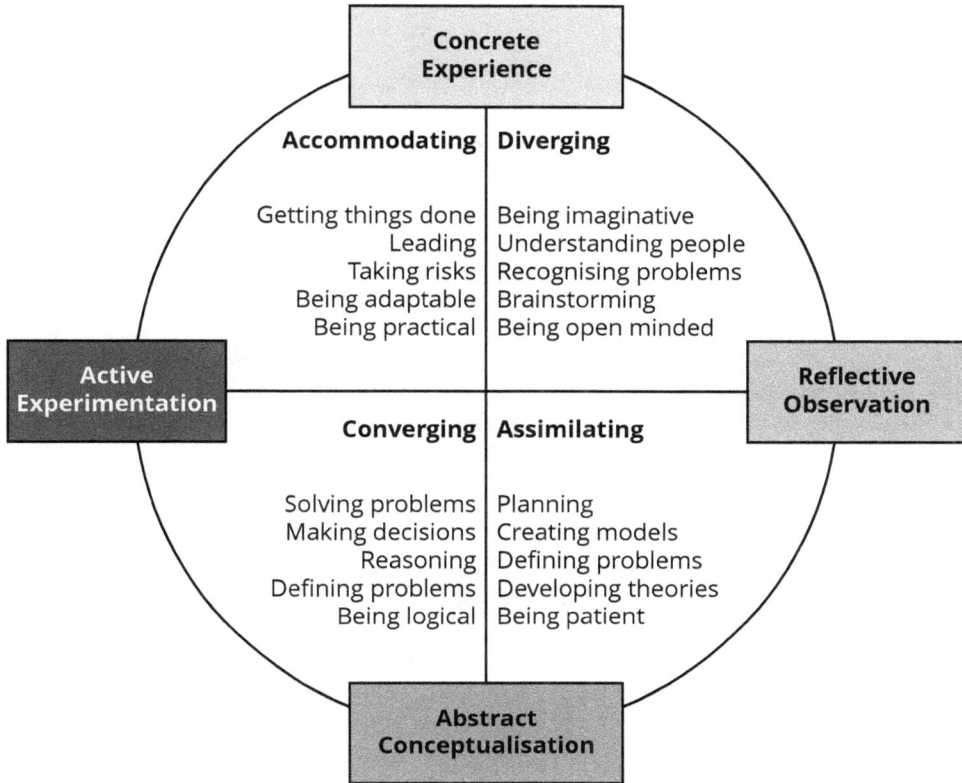

Figure 2.2   Kolb's learning cycle

Eyler (2018) discusses this in the context of 'service learning' by using learning experiences rather than learning information in isolation. In healthcare education, this is called application of theory in practice, and enables you to use that knowledge to apply to other new situations appropriately. This helps you to meet the NMC (2018a) The Code: Standards of professional behaviour for nurses, midwives and nursing associates, where knowledge is necessary for safe practice with the ability to evaluate the team's work to ensure practice is safe and effective. This requires you to give and receive feedback, reflect on that to improve your practice and manage any differences of opinion respectfully through discussion and debate. As you progress through the programme, you will start to support others in developing professional competence and confidence, stepping in where there is a likelihood for an error to occur based on knowledge and evidence, including the role that human or system error (also known as human factors) has. This requires self-awareness of your own behaviours and how these impact on others to allow you to identify learning opportunities that help you maintain and develop your competence to improve your practice.

Case study: Uchechi

Uchechi is from Nigeria, having settled in the UK several years ago. They have completed the 1st year of the SNA programme and are reflecting on this. This has been broken down to apply Kolb's experiential learning cycle.

(Continued)

23

(Continued)

I had an experience of learning on my student nursing associate course that I did not want to speak in class or share my ideas (Concrete Experience) as I was worried I may get it wrong, or that others may not understand my accent, so I sat and listened (Observation). The majority of the group were confident and spoke up, but I often felt they dominated the discussions with ideas that could be expanded and more inclusive of patients from different backgrounds (Diverging). I reflected on their ideas and my own ideas (Assimilating) to then think about what needed to change (Abstract Conceptualism). I then talked to the other students who were also under-represented in the group, to see what they thought (Converging). We decided that if we worked together, we could collectively expand the discussion without it falling onto one person to be 'brave'. We then started to add in our thoughts, one would start then another would add (Active Experimentation). As we got used to this, we felt more comfortable and confident in expressing our thoughts and ideas (Accommodating). This meant we were able to experience participating in class discussions (Concrete Experience).

One of the key features of Kolb's cycle is feelings related to the concrete experience. The case study started by identifying how Uchechi was worried about speaking up in class. We all have experiences and memories which have feelings attached to them. Making the association between your experiences and the feelings they created will help you start to identify when positive or negative feelings are having a positive or negative influence on your current learning. It is important to recognise that your previous experiences will influence your actions; therefore, gaining insight into the emotional response and then reflecting on why you feel that emotion can help identify alternative approaches. Kolb (2015) explored this by explaining we grasp understanding through apprehension (worry).

Activity 2.3   Reflection

Look at the following list of emotional feelings and related descriptors (González, 2013). Identify your own words that relate to each emotion and add them to the list:

- Fear: dread, cowardice, afraid, terrified, scared, scary, terrible.
- Rage: anger, wrath, angry.
- Love: desire, appetence, affection, attraction.
- Happiness: joy, delight, pleasure, happy.
- Sadness: sorrow, grief, affliction, sad, miserable.
- Shame: embarrassment, humiliation, shy.
- Pride: arrogance, proud.
- Fault: guilt, culpability, disappoint.
- Hope: confidence, confident, expectation.
- Sympathy: empathy, compassion, pity.
- Hate: aversion, dislike, disgust.

Take 5 minutes to identify which colour you relate to that emotion as this can help you visualise these before thinking about the following:

What is your most positive (or best) experience of learning?

Why was it good?

How did it make you feel?

Now think how you can link your current learning experiences to that positive experience. If you can do this, that positive emotional feeling will accompany the new learning experience. This will help improve how you feel, as your thoughts and feelings work together to help you engage with your learning, which will also support building your confidence with your studies. You could visualise these positive feelings with the colours that you associated with the emotion.

This activity is a personal reflection, so there is no outline answer at the end of the chapter.

Starting to reflect

When you break down the process of reflection, you can identify some key stages in this to enable you to extend your thinking. To start thinking about reflection, it is important to think about the process involved first.

Stage 1 Self-awareness and looking internally

Self-awareness and self-reflection are critical to professional development. This involves learning a new set of 'norms' and behaviours as part of your professional development. Looking at yourself is the first and most important stage, and receiving feedback will support or challenge your views of yourself.

Stage 2 How do others see me?

Consider how your peers see you through peer assessment, socialisation and ad-hoc feedback. In your classes, think about verbal and written feedback you have received or discussions with your tutors. Your supervisors' feedback in practice, both verbal and written feedback and assessment, will help you identify areas where you work well and areas you still need to develop. You will be required to gain service user feedback at all stages of your career; consider whether you should ask someone who you found it difficult to care for as they may be more likely to help you see what you do and how you do it, including what impact this had on their episode of care. It takes courage, one of the 6 Cs (explored in Chapter 5), to ask for honest feedback to improve your practice. Think back to Chapter 1 and the Johari Window – are there hidden areas that perhaps need to be revealed by you or shared with you that can enable you to continue to grow as a professional practitioner?

Putting stages 1 and 2 together, consider whether your view of yourself matches with the view of others. If not, ask yourself why, what are the differences and look at how these affect your behaviour. Then you can explore how this influences your development as a healthcare professional.

Stage 3 Confirming what you are learning from stages 1 and 2

You can use reflection on the outcomes of your actions to set learning goals. For example, you may decide to focus on a specific proficiency within the NMC (2024a) Standards, such as

1.15, take responsibility for continuous self-reflection, seeking and responding to support and feedback to develop professional knowledge and skills. Revisit Chapter 1 and SMART goals to ensure you create outcomes that you can clearly recognise as being achievable; for example, creation of a reflective journal in practice. You then have a clear outcome; completion of reflection within the reflective journal to measure the outcome. It is equally important to then work out why it worked, which links to the process of clinical reasoning, a skill that you need to cultivate across all your practice. Finally, you will need to judge how well you communicated to gain feedback and whether you approached and managed this in an objective way.

Models of reflection

Through exploring some different reflection models, you can see how these can be used to develop your own reflective practice. There are many different models available, but here we focus on the ones that are easy to use and understand, as they will help you with the first steps of formal reflection.

What, so what and now what

Borton's (1970) model is an example of how Kolb's framework of experiential learning has been developed to support the reflective process. This was more simplified in its approach: for example, 'What' is Kolb's *observation* stage; the question 'So What' is a prompt to theorise (to propose a reason) from the description, again, based on Kolb's *conceptualisation* stage. The 'Now What' stage is about thinking to the future to plan an action based on the previous stage and links to Kolb's *active experimentation* stage.

Activity 2.4   Critical thinking

What do you think the advantages of Borton's model are in comparison to Kolb's cycle?

What do you think some of the challenges of the model may be?

Outline answers at the end of the chapter.

Gibbs (1988)

Gibbs' model is popular with novice reflective practitioners as it has a simple set of headings and questions that prompt you to think about different parts of an experience, as it looks to pay attention to key parts of the reflective process (see Figure 2.3). First, describing your experience, exploring what you felt and thought at the time (Description and Feelings). Using Activity 2.3 can help you with the feeling part of Gibbs' cycle. The next stage involves evaluating what was good and bad about the situation to understand what happened and why (Evaluation and Analysis). Using critical thinking can help you to think about what else you could have done at the time, perhaps why you did not take that action and what the outcome may have been if you had (Conclusion). This is to help you think about what you may do differently in a similar situation. This presents an opportunity to create an action plan for you to follow next time (Action Plan).

Activity 2.5 Critical thinking

Thinking back to Chapter 1 and your action plan, what principles can you take to apply to create a reflective action plan?

This activity is a personal response, so there is no outline answer at the end of the chapter.

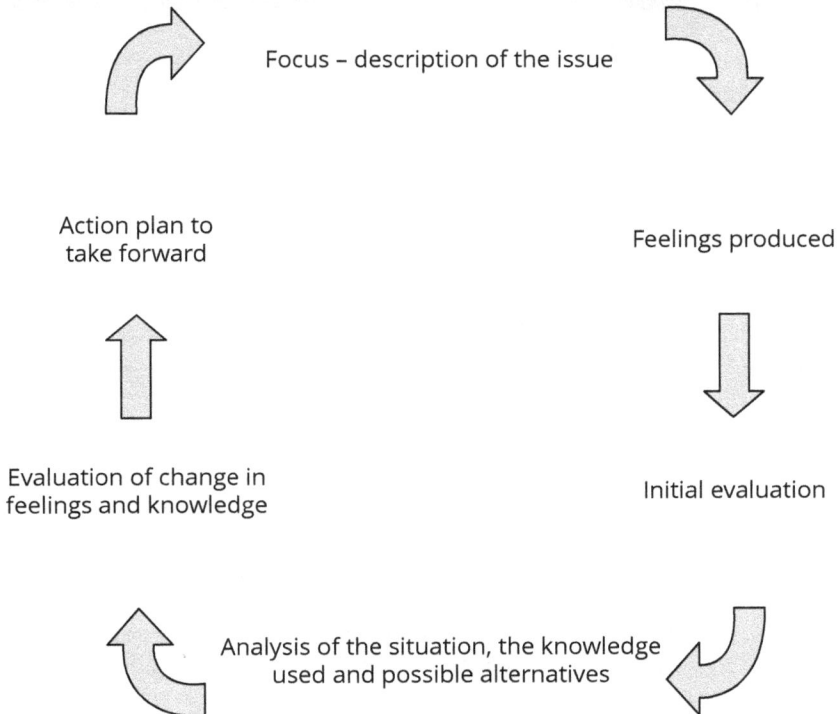

Focus – description of the issue

Action plan to
take forward

Feelings produced

Evaluation of change in
feelings and knowledge

Initial evaluation

Analysis of the situation, the knowledge
used and possible alternatives

Figure 2.3 Gibbs' (1988) cycle

One of the challenges you may find using Gibbs (1988) is that it is generic in the headings and, once completed, there is no indication on how the action plan links to description. It focuses on the evaluation of the experience, but does not get you to think about knowledge and how you use this to change what you do. As a novice reflective practitioner, it may be tempting to give a short outline for each section. However, consider the purpose of the model and how you can unpick why you felt the way you did, what shaped your thinking, what you know or have experienced before, as these all affect and shape the way you think and act. The action plan does create an opportunity to commit to changing your approach, but has been criticised for simplifying the action plan to an action you would do differently in future, as it lacks analysis of what impact those actions may have.

The important thing to remember with any reflective process is that these are tools that are designed to help you understand and learn from your experiences. As you progress through your studies, you will be able to use knowledge of theories to help shape your understanding and improve actions you take. As you become more familiar with reflection as an activity, you can experiment with different models to see which works well for you in different situations. The next section explores some more models that you may find useful when you reach that stage.

Activity 2.6 Reflection

Using Borton's reflective model, What, So what and Now what, reflect on a recent negative experience in practice.

Repeat the reflection using Gibbs' model.

Which did you find the easiest?

Why was it easier?

What did you learn from the experience?

This activity is a personal reflection, so there is no outline answer at the end of the chapter.

Rolfe (2001)

Rolfe (2001, cited in Rolfe et al. 2011, p. 45) expanded Bolton's framework in response to criticism that it does not outline some of the finer details required for reflective analysis and how this may be developed through each stage. This was achieved by adding some question points under each element of the cycle to stimulate greater depth of analysis (Table 2.1). This was designed as a non-specific (generic) framework to use for personal or group verbal and written reflections. The intention is that it can be used and adapted to meet your needs in different situations. The questions are to stimulate thinking but can be adapted to fit different experiences or situations. It is important to follow the sequence, so you follow the three steps in that order. The first time you reflect using the framework, you are mainly describing your experience, but you can return and then build on this to gain insight and understanding. The framework then becomes a cycle that can be repeated until you reach a deeper understanding through reflecting on your reflections. This cyclical process also helps you to 'think through' potential outcomes of future actions with the aim of bringing about change.

Table 2.1   Rolfe's (2001) framework

Descriptive level of reflection	Theory and knowledge building level of reflection	Action orientated (reflexive) level of reflection
What	So what	Now what
What is the problem/difficulty/ reason for being stuck/reason for feeling bad/reason we don't get on etc, etc? What was my role in the situation?	So what does this tell/teach me/ imply/mean about my patient/ professional relationship/model of care I am using/my attitudes/ my patients' attitudes/my colleagues' attitudes?	Now what do I need to do in order to make things better/stop being stuck/improve my patient's care/resolve the situation/feel better/get on better?

Descriptive level of reflection	Theory and knowledge building level of reflection	Action orientated (reflexive) level of reflection
What	**So what**	**Now what**
What was I trying to achieve?	So what was going through my mind as I acted?	Now what broader issues need to be considered if this action is to be successful?
What actions did I take?		
What was the response of others?	So what did I base my actions on?	Now what might be the consequences of this action?
What were the consequences	So what other knowledge can be brought to think about the situation:	
For the patient?		
For myself?	Factual?	
For others?	Professional?	
What feelings did it evoke	Personal?	
In the patient?	So what could/should I have done to make it better?	
In myself?		
In others?	So what are the broader issues that arose/that may arise from the situation?	
What was good/bad about the experience?		

Over time, your skills using formal or structured reflection will develop and you will find different reflective models less, or more useful, to the process. There are many models, so when you become proficient with this you can start to explore some of the more complex concepts of reflection, such as **reflexivity**. Reflexivity moves from doing a piece of reflection, to incorporating some critical thinking about your own responses, interaction and outcomes to create a personal **perspective** of what happened, why it happened and what other actions may have changed the outcome, and what those outcomes could be in future if different actions are taken. Being reflexive is the outcome of Rolfe's framework of repeatedly reflecting on your reflection. Level 1 is your descriptive reflection, which as a novice reflective practitioner may be initially where you are reflecting. Level 2 is when you can think about how and why this situation occurred in the first place, for example, linking to theory and previous experiences and/or knowledge you have. Level 3 moves forward through a deliberate return to reflect on level 2 and intends to change to improve. It is at this point you are developing a reflexive approach. This shifts the focus from rational-based knowledge to using your knowledge and experience (professional artistry) to incorporate strong criticality. This is more about who you are and what you do through increased self-awareness, increased critical thinking and moves from doing reflection towards being reflective within your practice to reflect-in-action rather than reflection-on-action.

Activity 2.7   Critical thinking

Repeat the reflection you completed in Activity 2.6 using Rolfe's model of reflection.

Did this create more challenges for you? Why?

Did you learn anything more about yourself or the situation you experienced by exploring in greater depth and detail through repeating the process?

This activity is a personal activity, so there is no outline answer at the end of the chapter.

Reflection-in-action and reflection-on-action (Schön, 1983; 1987)

Reflection-on-action is the process of looking back at an event and analysing it to make explicit the knowledge which guided action.

Reflection-in-action is the process of thinking about and altering action during an experience. The process is usually employed when faced with an unexpected event.

Schön acknowledged that reflection is looking back on your experience as a way of thinking and understanding it. He termed this *Reflection-on-action* and this is used extensively in education of healthcare practitioners. He then explored *Reflection-in-action* to think about an experience in the moment. This allows you to identify that something requires an immediate change, readjusting an action to account for unexpected obstacles or influences. This may need you to stop and think in the moment, or you may recognise and adjust actions seamlessly based on experience and knowledge to demonstrate problem-solving, while understanding that the previous way of thinking is not enough.

This **research**-based theory has been used to explore rationale-based knowledge, and professional artistry, which is defined as knowing-in-action. Although both types of knowledge are necessary in professional healthcare practice, Schön believed professional artistry holds more significance as you need to know how to respond to everyday situations in practice. This does require technical, or rationale-based knowledge to inform the clinical decisions you make; however, these are taken together with knowledge from your previous experiences. Each experience, however, will be unique to the individual involved and the context or situation, so although there may be similarities, you need to be able to adapt your responses as events unfold for the specific situation you are faced with. These differences may be subtle, and you will need to be able to appreciate this requires you to understand less obvious forms of knowledge, such as intuition. For example, you may sense something is not right, but may be unable to articulate what is wrong, why it is wrong or why you responded the way you did. Intuition in professional practice is considered tacit knowledge, or knowledge understood or implied. By exploring these experiences through storytelling, you can build a picture of what you know or understand about the situation to try and focus on the whole scenario. This makes you central to the experience rather than external to it, with reflexivity as an important part of this process.

Identify which of these models you feel most comfortable using. One aspect of professional practice required by the NMC is reflection on practice to create new knowledge and learning. According to the NMC (2019a), the benefits of professionals' continued reflective practice facilitates better patient experiences, particularly when practitioners reflect together. There are challenges to group reflections that you may experience, so it can be helpful to start reflecting with someone you feel comfortable with. The importance of openness and honesty in reflection cannot be emphasised enough, but you may want to reflect privately before you first reflect with someone else. This can help you feel confident in your thoughts and feelings before you start a reflection with another person. Many practitioners keep a reflective journal where they regularly reflect on their experiences. These are useful tools in learning, as you will be able to try and use this on experiences from practice to help you develop this skill. It can also be helpful to support your academic work as you can show how you apply learning in practice to what you have learnt in class. As you develop proficiency with reflection you can start to deepen this further still with reflexivity, as discussed earlier, to then start to consider reflection in, as well as on, action.

Unconscious bias

The role of unconscious bias is an important consideration in any reflective activity you undertake in practice and in your academic learning. We all have bias, but can you identify your own bias? It is actually quite difficult as the fundamental processes involve assessment and judgement which use autonomic (unconscious) reflexes of stress (watch the TED talk by Valerie Alexander listed in the annotated reading for more detailed information). These assessments and judgements are formed through our background, personal experience, cultural and social influences, such as what we consider acceptable or normal.

A stressful situation, whether caused by the environment, such as a looming assignment deadline, or psychological, such as worrying about work, triggers stress hormones that produce physiological changes. A stressful experience can cause the heart to pound, breathing to quicken, tensing of muscles or sweating. This combination of reactions to stress is also known as the 'fight-or-flight' response, originally intended as a survival mechanism, enabling people to react quickly to life-threatening situations. The near-instant hormonal changes and physiological responses aim to fight off the threat or flee to safety. Today, we are faced with few real life-threatening situations, so your body can now also overreact to stressors that are not life-threatening, such as traffic jams, work pressure, family difficulties or situations that you feel uncertain or unsafe in for a whole range of reasons.

One aspect of reflection can be to recognise your own feelings and responses to a situation that may have negatively impacted, either for you or on the outcome of the situation. Being aware of beliefs and values that you hold strongly, and recognising how and when these may influence your attitudes and approaches in situations, is an important element of reflexivity. You are a unique individual, with experiences spanning your life that influence your attitudes and behaviours. You may not always be aware that these may have a negative impact at times, sometimes through a negative thought or feeling, but also through feeling positive towards a particular group of people to favour them over others. For example, as a woman, you may feel more comfortable in talking to women to help them express their needs, whereas with men, your experience has been they 'get on with it' and tend not to open-up about things they struggle with. This may mean you give greater time and utilise your communication skills more effectively with women compared to men. One basic way of checking whether you have a different attitude towards a group of people is to ask yourself, would I repeat this action/approach in the same way with a different group. This could be based on gender, sexuality, age, religion, disability, culture or race to name a few. The key is to analyse why you felt that way and what you need to do to shift your thinking.

Activity 2.8   Reflection

What bias are you aware of having?

What bias are you aware of others you know well of having?

What indicators have you had that may identify these?

Do you think they are aware of them?

If not, how comfortable would you feel in telling them?

Now apply this to practice – people you work with in the team *and* patients – they too have bias.

Reflect for a moment on the impact your own bias may have on the way you behave or respond to a situation that encompasses that bias. Remember, this is a bias you are aware of. Now think about how you react and respond negatively in situations; try using a reflective model to unpick what influenced your reaction and response; is there something in your life experience,

(Continued)

(Continued)

the way you were brought up or your beliefs and values that has unduly influenced your actions in a negative way? Now think about that reaction, what impact did it have on other person/people involved? What could you do to think about your reaction differently so you can respond in a way that is less harmful to the situation?

This activity is a personal reflection, so there is no outline answer at the end of the chapter.

The NMC (2021) recognises that bias is a major influence on who gets referred to them for fitness to practise concerns and highlights that any bias identified in a referral is taken seriously and they will explore that to ensure discrimination is not playing a part. The *Standards of Proficiency for Nursing Associates* (NMC, 2024a) also have specific proficiencies that relate to bias 1.3, 1.4, 1.11 and a range of others that link to related skills that demonstrate understanding your own approaches and the impact these may have on others.

Chapter summary

This chapter has explored the role of reflection to highlight as an essential skill for nursing associate practice to meet the requirements of the NMC (2024a). Essentially, you need to think of the experience as a learning opportunity; an opportunity to learn something about yourself and how you approach your work, both academic and practice based. If you find reflection or using these models challenging, then it can be helpful to talk to your registered colleagues as they will be experienced in using this both within learning, in practice and for revalidation of their registration with the NMC. Using a structured model such as Rolfe or Gibbs can help you when you are starting out, but as a novice reflective practitioner, it may take you time to develop the skills to deepen your understanding. Over time, reflecting on your reflections can enable you to learn more about yourself and the how and why situations occurred, to lead you to a deeper understanding for future change. Exploring your own attitudes, beliefs and values is a key step in creating fair and equitable approaches to the care you give to all those you work with and care for within the practice environment.

Activities: Brief outline answers

Activity 2.1 Reflection (page 20)

Does this have different meanings for you in different places and at different times? *Here you may have considered experiences where you see a physical reflection in a mirror or in water; this shows the image but reversed, so you do not see this exactly as it appears – which many people fail to recognise. This helps you to consider the different perspectives that reflection can give.*

Why do you reflect?

Here you may have thought about reflection as a way of thinking about something – a problem or an experience that you want to understand, or perhaps you use this when making decisions in your life.

When do you consciously reflect?

When you consciously reflect, you are thinking about a specific experience, situation or event; for example, why did I do that, how did I do that, what options are there. These are all examples of when you consciously reflect.

How do you consciously reflect?

Some of you will consciously reflect when talking to others about a situation, offering reasons why something happened or how you need to approach something. You may have consciously reflected in practice, for example, following a critical incident or a near miss. You may use a model already or you may just take time to write the experience down. Usually, you would have to make time to consciously reflect.

Activity 2.2 Reflection in practice (page 22)

What are your experiences of reflection in practice?

Here you may have identified debrief following a near miss or critical incident, or you may already be using a reflective journal.

Have you reflected with other people?

Chatting with colleagues about what happened is a form of informal reflection, whereas a debrief is often a structured experience. Consider whether you felt safe reflecting with others or whether you spent time reflecting first; or possibly listening to what others had to say before deciding what to share with them.

Do you reflect regularly on your actions?

You may or may not reflect regularly but it is important to think about the art of reflection, taking time and practice to achieve meaningful reflection for professional practice.

Do you only reflect when something has not gone to plan?

This is a common experience but there are important lessons to learn from positive experiences so you can utilise those in future too.

Do you write down your reflections?

You may find it difficult to find time to write reflections down when you are trying to balance your studies, demands of work and family commitments. Even if you only write one reflection a month, it is a good starting point. Certainly, while you are completing the nursing associate programme, you will be expected to reflect on practice in your practice assessment documents. Make sure you give yourself time to complete these as they are an excellent source of evidence of your professional growth to help and support you throughout your studies and beyond.

Activity 2.4 Critical thinking (page 26)

What do you think the advantages of Borton's model are in comparison to Kolb's cycle? *It is easy to complete without requiring reminder of what is needed. This can work well for early reflective practice.*

Challenges of the model? *This is a simple model, which possibly misses finer details of reflection as does not prompt in-depth analysis.*

Annotated further reading

Mahon, P. and O'Neill, M. (2020) 'Through the looking glass: the rabbit hole of reflective practice', *British Journal of Nursing*, 29(13), pp. 777–783. doi:10.12968/bjon.2020. 29.13.777.

This article explores the role of reflection and the impact of unconscious bias to highlight the implications of this. They question whether and how reflection addresses unconscious biases as these are relatively unexplored in the nursing literature. The role of accurate self-assessment in successful reflective practice, and the potential impact of unconscious bias on reflection, are discussed in some depth. The authors conclude that while biases may limit our ability to learn from reflection, therefore, this is even more reason to critically engage with the process.

NMC (2019d) *Regulators unite to support reflective practice across health and care.* www.nmc.org.uk/news/press-releases/joint-statement-reflective-practice/

The NMC states that 'Reflection is how health and care professionals can assess their professional experiences – both positive and where improvements may be needed – recording and documenting insight to aid their learning and identify opportunities to improve.

Reflection allows an individual to continually improve the quality of care they provide and gives multi-disciplinary teams the opportunity to reflect and discuss openly and honestly.'

NMC (2021) *Ensuring your decisions to refer are fair and unbiased.* www.nmc.org.uk/ employer-resource/deciding-to-refer/fair-unbiased-decisions/ This explores how the NMC view biased referrals for fitness to practice and links to their own research on how different groups are adversely affected by biased referrals.

How to Outsmart Your Own Unconscious Bias. www.youtube.com/watch?v=GP-cqFLS8Q4 In this video, Valerie Alexander explains the physiological responses to stress.

Chapter 3

Resilience for professional practice

NMC (2024A) *STANDARDS OF PROFICIENCY FOR NURSING ASSOCIATES*

This chapter will address the following platforms and proficiencies.

Platform 1: Being an accountable professional

1.1   Understand and act in accordance with The Code: Professional standards of practice and behaviour for nurses, midwives and nursing associates, and fulfil all registration requirements.

1.5   Understand the demands of professional practice and demonstrate how to recognise signs of vulnerability in themselves or their colleagues and the action required to minimise risks to health.

1.8   Understand and explain the meaning of resilience and emotional intelligence, and their influence on an individual's ability to provide care.

1.10 Demonstrate the skills and abilities required to develop, manage and maintain appropriate relationships with people, their families, carers and colleagues.

Platform 2: Promoting health and preventing ill health

2.5   Understand the importance of early years and childhood experiences and the possible impact on life choices, mental, physical and behavioural health and well-being.

Platform 5: Improving safety and quality of care

5.9   Recognise uncertainty and demonstrate an awareness of strategies to develop resilience in themselves. Know how to seek support to help deal with uncertain situations.

Chapter aims

- Explore the role of resilience and how this influences professional practice.
- Consider how to develop and maintain professional resilience.
- Identify the role of professional resilience in leadership in practice.
- Outline organisational resilience and the impact this has on the health and care workforce.

Introduction

This chapter follows on from Chapter 2 discussions on reflection, reflexivity and self-awareness to consider how these support self-management and resilience, both personally and professionally. You will explore the concept of resilience, the impact personal and professional challenges have, and how these impact each other. The psychological basis of stress will be outlined to enable recognition of your own signs and symptoms of this, linking it to the impact that the expectations we set ourselves can have. This relates to **emotional intelligence**, the ability to recognise both our own and others' emotional state, which can impact care giving. The role of burnout, coping with demanding work and workloads, and experience of systemic barriers for minority groups, such as people from ethnic minority backgrounds, cultural differences, or neurodiversity, will link to self-care and the importance of managing your own mental and physical health for well-being. You will consider how to manage your own needs to be resilient with the help of the role played by support networks, Schwartz Rounds (Golding, 2024) and mindfulness. The role of organisational resilience will be explored to see how you may be affected by this.

Background

When you work in a caring profession, whether you are based in a hospital, General Practitioner (GP) practice, care home, working in patients' homes, a prison healthcare facility or other health provision, you will be faced with being available to your patients, service users or clients, often at times of vulnerability. People need you to be there for them, to help them navigate or manage the care system, their health needs or other wide-ranging needs. You, as a nursing associate or student nursing associate, have made a commitment to support people in meeting their care needs to meet the NMC (2024a) *Standards of Proficiency for Nursing Associates* and the NMC (2018a) *The Code: Standards of Professional Behaviour.* You will stand by their side, hold their hand, be a form of gentle support, offering a skilful presence to reassure, ease discomfort and re-establish well-being. These are undertaken mindfully, with awareness of the responsibility you have to your patient, but at times, they can take their toll on your own emotional well-being, particularly when you are faced with additional stressors within your own life. This can include undertaking a programme of study, as discussed in Chapter 1 – balancing your own needs, your family commitments and the need to work on top of having enough time to study and complete assessment is demanding. Life has a nasty habit of sneaking up on you when you least expect it, and how you manage and cope with those unexpected, or even expected events, can cause difficulties in managing your emotional health and well-being.

What is resilience?

Resilience has several definitions, depending on the point of view being looked at. It can be your capacity to tolerate excessive demands and stressors without experiencing stress-related problems that affect your performance; for example, managing assignments while working and supporting your family's needs. It can also be determination to see something through, such as when you find it difficult on a placement, you make the most of the learning opportunity despite the challenges; or an ability to 'bounce back' from a challenging situation to continue as you usually would, such as at the end of a stressful time in a personal relationship that resulted in being less focused on an assignment; you are able to pick this up again once the relationship issue is resolved. Therefore, this can be thought of as a process (working through the issue to manage your needs), an outcome (being resilient as a result of the issue after it is resolved) and an ability (able to manage the issue without it affecting you unduly) (Southwick et al., 2016).

Case study: Andreia

Resilience as a process: Andreia settled in the UK after being displaced from Ukraine due to the conflict. Unfortunately, their family were not all able to leave so they have been unable to spend time together, but Andriea talks a lot about their 'UK family' who offered a home and have become their main source of social support. Andreia spent time studying English to be able to gain a qualification and contribute to the society that had offered refuge during the conflict. At home, they were employed in the leisure industry but felt that they needed to be able to make a significant contribution to the hosting society that could also support their homeland, should they ever be able to return. They were able to secure a role as a healthcare assistant at a local care home and offered the opportunity to complete the nursing associate course as an apprenticeship.

Resilience as an outcome: Andreia has been in the UK and studying hard for three years now, coming towards the end of the SNA course. They have struggled with English not being their first language, as well as academic study, which they had not attempted before. They spoke to their personal tutor who suggested they access the academic student support but there have been times when Andreia has been deeply frustrated and upset. The final straw came when their brother was injured because of the conflict at home, which resulted in taking some time out from studying. Having six months away has enabled Andreia to refocus following their brother's recovery and they have now returned with renewed determination.

Resilience as an ability: Andreia recognised the strategies that helped them to manage overcome this experience and so, in the following assessment period, they accessed support from student services, tutors, their peers and their 'UK family'. Putting these strategies in place helped Andreia successfully complete the assessments without feeling overwhelmed and stressed as they had previously.

Resilience as an outcome: Andreia's self-awareness, and ability to seek support when needed, helped them to manage their needs at different times which result in managing these effectively.

The passion, determination and perseverance you have for achieving your long-term goals has been referred to as 'grit' (Duckworth, 2016) and this has been shown to determine academic and professional success regardless of your IQ (intelligence quotient), which measures human intelligence, including your ability to resolve or solve problems; therefore, determination to succeed involves resolving or solving problems you encounter along the way.

Activity 3.1   Reflection

Reflect on an experience where you had a negative emotional reaction to change within your practice as a student nursing associate (SNA)/nursing associate (NA).

Now reflect on an experience where you were resilient when faced with a change in practice.

Consider why you reacted differently in the two situations.

Can you identify the three different types of resilience through your experiences?

(Continued)

(Continued)

Was this a resilient process?

Was resilience the outcome?

Do you feel your resilience is an ability?

This activity is a personal reflection, so the outline answer at the end of the chapter provides guidance only.

Resilience in individuals is needed to manage risks arising from life events that may include challenges or threats to health and well-being. The NMC (2024a) *Standards of Proficiency for Nursing Associates* recognise the importance of managing your own emotional health and well-being, including vulnerability in yourself and other colleagues; therefore, it is important that you can explore your own emotional well-being needs. To assist you in developing a theoretical understanding, a conceptual framework, Neuman Systems Model (1995 cited in Turner and Kaylor, 2015), which focuses on humans, environment, health and nursing, will be used to explore resilience within health and care settings. Later in the chapter, we will describe strategies that help promote resilience development in nursing.

Understanding theory

Neuman developed an approach to think about resilience within the nursing profession as they recognised that by keeping nurses emotionally resilient, the impact on patient care and healing could be strengthened through reducing the patient experience of stress. The basis of the model considers that patients interact within an environment, continuously responding to changes within this. To enable this to happen, patients develop strategies to defend themselves from stressors that may result in a positive or negative outcome. This ability to adjust and adapt to the environment is a normal defence process, which results in the patient's wellness level being maintained, described as a 'protective buffer,' as it prevents stressors overwhelming normal well-being levels. The role of social support, spirituality and a person's age are recognised as being key areas for maintaining status quo of well-being.

When this defence mechanism is challenged with environmental stressors, the patient has an adverse response. Your response can help in a few ways, with an initial intervention, such as identifying risk factors or using a health promotion approach. The next line of support could include trying to expand the patient's defence system through actions that strengthen this, for example, active listening, meditation or mindfulness activities.

One of the challenges recognised within Neuman's Systems Model (1995) is the role of physiological, psychological, sociocultural, developmental and spiritual elements that must be considered. Understanding the physiological response to stress, as discussed in Chapter 2, will help you understand your patient's responses to stress; stress hormones produce physiological changes that cause the heart to pound, breathing to quicken, tensing of muscles or sweating, the 'fight-or-flight' response. This requires an understanding of the patient themselves and their unique life experiences, beliefs and values, and will require you to keep an open mind to why they are reacting the way they are. You need to remember that being in a care environment removes patients from their normal environment. This interrupts basic routines and removes autonomy to make decisions, such as what to wear, what to eat and who they are sharing the space with. This can be disempowering for patients and create stress and vulnerability where it does not usually exist in addition to the ill-health experience that resulted in needing to access a health service.

Once you have acquired skills in recognising the patient's responses to stressors in the care environment, it is important that you consider your own reactions and responses to these. You will face stressors within the care environment as well; demands on managing your workload, staff sickness, patients deteriorating, relatives visiting and wanting information, as well as meeting your own basic needs for hydration, nutrition or elimination, which may need to wait because of the demands being made on your time. These may be on top of personal stressors, such as managing your home and family, ill-health within the family, demands others may make on you, and of course, the requirements to complete your studies. These impact in your ability to manage your own responses to stressors and can result in not maintaining positive emotional well-being.

Underpinning resilience

When you think about your own responses to stressors, it may help if you understand some of the underpinning processes that enable or hinder these to manage the NMC (2024a) requirements within the nursing associate standards.

Biological, personality and sociocultural connections

The biological impact of hormones and autonomic nervous system is linked to the ability to cope with stress. Some people's personality may exhibit defiance, or they may be a risk taker or an optimist, and these may change at different ages and stages of life. This is because your brain continues to develop and change throughout your life; for example, executive function (the ability to control and manage your thoughts and behaviour) and social cognition (thinking). In parts of the brain of younger people, there is increased amounts of white matter where decision-making takes place and reduction in grey matter, where understanding the risk to themselves and understanding others' perspectives is underdeveloped. These differ across genders but have been linked to development of mental health issues across adolescence (Schweizer et al., 2023). This links to sociocultural perspectives, as life experiences can influence how you deal with situations and your coping strategies. The support that you have around you can influence how you will deal with a situation. Therefore, it is important for you to recognise how your age can influence your experience, how you manage your emotional needs and the influence on decisions you make in those moments. This relates to NMC (2024a). Requirement to understand resilience and emotional intelligence, and how this influences your ability to provide care.

What determines resilience?

Various factors underpin resilience as explored below.

Activity 3.2   Reflection

What things do you think you need to be a resilient person both professionally and privately?

This activity is a personal reflection, so the outline answer at the end of the chapter provides guidance only.

Self-mastery

Your outlook on life and how you view yourself and others will be influenced by your upbringing and environment. When facing adverse situations, a positive outlook has been found to result in stronger coping behaviours to protect and result in a quicker recovery. This helps to improve your health and well-being, and achieve a sense of self-mastery. Conversely, a negative view of yourself and others can increase how you perceive stress, and limit your self-mastery and belief that you can manage the challenges you face. Therefore, if you see things negatively, you are more likely to think narrowly, have limited belief in yourself and negative self-talk that can result in less effective coping habits.

Social support

Support comes in the form of family, intimate partners, colleagues, neighbours, friends and spiritual community members, to name a few. Strong support networks and using social support are linked with resilience, as they strengthen the ability to endure psychological challenges. It has been shown that better quality of life results from strong social bonds, and for your patients, wound healing, and life expectancy are also positively influenced. In contrast, a weaker sense of control and depression are associated with a lack of support.

As a resilient person, you will develop the ability to communicate effectively, creating healthy social bonds and show value and compassion. These are traits that enable you to be an effective nursing associate and meet the NMC *Standards of Proficiency for Nursing* Associates (2024a). It is important to recognise that you can learn to improve your ability to form healthier relationships and stronger networks of support.

A myriad of traits is associated with a positive outlook. Those most associated with resilience are believing that success is possible (optimism), viewing difficulties as opportunities for growth and learning, having the willingness to push forward, being able to accept change, and being open to making mistakes and learning from failures. All these traits can be cultivated with practice and are not dependent on upbringing and genetics.

Genes

A range of genes has been identified that are associated with resilient phenotypes (how a gene expresses itself physically). Various genes have been identified that influence responses to stress, the role of the nervous and immune systems, as well as production of serotonin and dopamine, neurotransmitters which decide your biological response to stress. Although science shows genes have a role in resilience, these can be influenced through life experience, as the role of nature and nurture work together. Therefore, self-mastery and social support can influence your genes in responding to stress.

Child development

Attachment theory (Bowlby, 1988) identified that a safe base and early childhood experiences can positively or negatively affect the development of the stress response and how individuals subsequently learn to cope with adversity. The central nervous system circuits are affected by trauma and abuse through a hyperactive stress response. This leads to more anxious behaviour, with helplessness being learnt as a belief that you cannot control adverse situations. When individuals realise changing behaviours is possible, the learnt helplessness does not occur. This knowledge helps understanding the importance of early years and childhood experiences and their possible impact on life choices, mental, physical and behavioural health and well-being outlined in the NMC (2024a) standards.

Cultural beliefs, values and expected behaviour can influence individual behaviour and coping styles. How you see yourself and your relationship with others may predict resilience; for example, the culture within your family will have influenced your own self-esteem and self-worth. It is important to remember that culture is not an ethnicity or religion but the attitudes of your family, friends and social network in which you were brought up. Cultures with strong core values that respectfully collaborate with open communication, have been shown to have strong resilience within the community as well as individual resilience.

Managing stress

You will have coping strategies that help you cope with stress; however, some of these may be maladaptive or adaptive. Maladaptive strategies may reduce feelings of anxiety and help you cope in the moment, but these are not healthy for your body; for example, smoking. Adaptive behaviours, therefore, are behaviours that help you cope with stress but are also positive healthy strategies that do not adversely affect your body or mind, for example going for a walk to clear your head.

Becoming more resilient

It is important that you are honest with yourself and realistic about what you can take on and manage effectively. There will be times when additional stressors impact on you; therefore, thinking about your own fears and confronting these head on, appraising situations realistically, calming your emotional responses and maintaining health behaviours, such as good sleep hygiene, and having a balanced nutritional input and exercise routine are all examples of adaptive coping habits.

Avoidance of managing your fears through immersing yourself in work, drinking alcohol or binge eating can all impact on your sleep, reduce your energy levels so you feel unable to exercise and are maladaptive coping habits.

There are some adaptive coping habits that can improve your resilience, such as meditation, yoga, accessing social support, connecting with your spiritual needs, reflecting on your thoughts and beliefs, regulating your emotions. Humour and laughter are good sources of coping with difficult experiences as they relieve the emotional burden and, psychologically, they relax your stress response. They have been shown to increase immune responses, reduce experience of pain, give you greater energy, as well as soothe tensions to improve your mood and increase your sense of well-being.

Spirituality is another important consideration. As previously discussed, this is not confined to religious or cultural beliefs but is an internal process that creates your values, ethical beliefs and social behaviours. If you have a strong sense of purpose, feel connected with your wider environment, this can enable management of traumatic events. Conversely, low spirituality is related to low resilience.

By developing and maintaining good relationships and support networks, accepting that some things cannot be changed, engaging in discovering yourself, thinking about the long term so that you do not make rash decisions and take care of your mind and body through good sleeping, eating and exercising habits, you will enhance your resilience and this will contribute to stronger self-confidence too, although some of these are easier than others and some are easier said than done!

You can develop greater awareness through mindfulness as this strengthens mastery through your immersion in the present moment. This involves you being able to observe your thoughts and emotions without becoming them. Some mindfulness exercises use colouring, but this can be any activity that requires you to give it your full attention, such as knitting or participating in a physical activity that you need to concentrate on.

For those with greater complex or distressing thoughts or emotions, cognitive behaviour therapy can help you learn to regulate your negative thoughts and memories, rather than getting stuck within them. This would require accessing professional support, either through your employer's occupational health service, your GP or student services where you are studying. In doing so, you would show that you recognise uncertainty and demonstrate an awareness of strategies to develop resilience in yourself, as required for NMC (2024a).

As discussed earlier, humour and laughter can be powerful tools to enable feeling less stressed as laughter can bring you into the present moment, difficult thoughts are left behind and future anxieties are not yet recognised. You can be distracted in a positive way, it can create intrigue, you want to find out what is so funny. This helps stop your mind focusing on the negative thoughts, breaking habits involved with patterns of negative thinking, inter-rupting the neural pathways to create new ones that are more positive, and laughter brings joy into your life (Neal and Gonot-Schoupinsky, 2023).

Maintaining balance

When it comes to the human brain, the ability to effectively multitask is a myth. Although computers can run two or more programs simultaneously, our brains must task-switch, and in the transfer of attention, time and productivity are lost. Monotasking, or single tasking, is now considered a way to increase productivity and actually maximise time. Evidence suggests that although you may feel that you manage a number of tasks at the same time, these will not be completed as well as they could be if completed individually. If you prioritise tasks at the start of the day, block calendar time to work on specific projects, pace yourself by scheduling rest periods, you can focus on one task and see this through to completion (Christensen, 2020).

Activity 3.3   Work-based learning

Use the questions below to evaluate how you approach managing your time and how suc-cessful you are with managing all you set out to achieve.

Track your week to evaluate how many individual tasks you have to manage.

Do you give your full attention to each task? If not, how many tasks are you trying to manage at the same time?

Are you experiencing aches, feeling stressed or out of rhythm with your life? If so, which tasks or demands are contributing to this?

Are you sleeping well, getting to sleep easily or managing to stay asleep? If not, what thoughts do you have when trying to sleep – do they relate to the demands you have?

Are you reflecting on your life experiences? If so, have you managed to identify what helps or hinders you?

Do you feel able to say no when you have a lot of conflicting demands on your time? What prevents you from saying no?

When you have completed this activity, reflect on your responses; do you need to work on managing your time to enable you to complete one task at a time?

Do you have any intrusive negative thinking that can benefit from using laughter or mindfulness approaches to create new thinking habits?

This activity is a personal reflection, so there is no outline answer at the end of the chapter.

Developing and maintaining resilience

Activity 3.4 Reflection

Can you identify any ways that you can monotask?

This activity is a personal reflection, so the outline answer at the end of the chapter provides guidance only.

	Self	Social
	1 Self-awareness	**3 Social-awareness**
Recognition of	Emotional Intelligence Accurate self-assessment Self confidence	Empathy Organisational awareness Understanding the service
	2 Self-management	**4 Relationship management**
Regulation through	Self-control Transparency Adaptability Initiative Achievement drive	Conflict management Building bonds and collaboration Change catalyst Teamwork and inspiring others Leadership and developing others

Figure 3.1 Goleman's emotional intelligence model adapted (2002)

Understanding theory

Goleman's (2020) Emotional Intelligence Model.

Goleman identified that emotional intelligence is how you manage yourself within your relationships through four areas, as seen in Figure 3.1:

(Continued)

(Continued)

1. self-awareness, knowing what you feel and why you feel that way, which are associated with positive decision-making;

2. self-management, which is how you manage your difficult emotional responses, so they do not hinder what you want or need to do, being able to adjust these so you are able to learn as all emotions have functions;

3. social-awareness, is having empathy, which is understanding how others feel and relating to that; and finally,

4. relationship management, how you put these together within your relationships.

Goleman argues that the area of the brain that governs emotional intelligence is the last part of the brain to develop; therefore, it is important to teach this to children so that, over time, they develop this skill. This does not mean that as an adult you are unable to learn and develop emotional intelligence; neuroplasticity of the brain continues throughout life and as you work on the different domains, you strengthen and develop the skills necessary for good emotional intelligence.

In being able to explore Goleman's model, you will support demonstration of skills and abilities required to develop, manage and maintain appropriate relationships with people, their families, carers and colleagues as identified within the NMC (2024a) standards.

Organisational resilience and the workforce

Goleman's work has focused on **leadership** in organisations, recognising the impact a leader's resilience has on those they lead and manage; therefore, it is not just you as an individual that requires the ability to be resilient. Good resilience within an organisation is necessary to manage risks; for example, during changes within the organisation, changes in the economic environment that impact on provision of services, political changes that influence policy directions within services, and staffing changes, such as being able to meet the provision of services. If an organisation lacks resilience, there is a risk to its reputation, as well as its ability to provide and maintain effective services. It is particularly important within care services as resilience in the workforce is needed to ensure their performance is maintained in service provision (Belasen, 2021).

Activity 3.5   Work-based learning

What factors may impact your organisation in terms of its resilience?

What factors impact staff resilience?

An outline answer is provided at the end of the chapter, but remember that each situation is different, so your experience in clinical practice may differ.

One initiative that has been developed within health and care services to enable staff resilience is Schwartz Rounds (Golding, 2024). This is a structured forum for staff across an organisation, whether providing frontline care or not, to provide a regular opportunity to come together and talk about the emotional and social experiences of working in healthcare. It aims to help you understand the challenges you experience, but also recognise the rewards of providing care. It does not intend to solve problems or focus solely on the clinical perspective of care provision, as it intends to support people in their roles through giving time and space to reflect on these. Evaluation of Schwartz Rounds has demonstrated that those who participate feel less stressed and isolated within their role and have a greater awareness and appreciation of others' roles. This can help to reduce the hierarchical nature between different roles, and the resulting increased compassion shown can also have a positive impact on patients' experiences of care. Participating in Schwartz Rounds can help demonstrate the NMC (2024a) standards highlighted at the start of the chapter.

Activity 3.6   Critical thinking

What do you think the challenges are for staff to participate in Schwartz Rounds?

An outline answer is provided at the end of the chapter.

Case study: Manuel

Manuel is participating in their first Schwartz Round on Imposter Syndrome at university. While listening to the three story tellers, they recognise some of the experiences, emotions and responses to situations, that although are not their experience, are similar. They grew up in a remote environment, kept away from school by their family. Throughout their childhood, they shared care responsibilities for their older sibling who had a learning disability and lacked opportunities to interact with other children. Since they have grown up, their sibling has died and they were left wondering what to do with their life, so they embarked on a distance learning programme during the pandemic and, subsequently, they moved to the local town and started working as a carer. Since then, they have moved further away from their family and entered other care environments, so when the student nursing associate opportunity presented itself, they felt they could apply for this. They have now been on the programme for four months. When the panel finished, the audience was invited to share their responses and experiences. After listening to others sharing their experiences, Manuel decides to speak up about their experience. Here they outline their childhood experience and share the challenges they have experienced being at university as a result. That they felt they do not belong and are not good enough, as they have not had any previous formal education, and socially, they feel awkward, not knowing the social cues for interaction with peers.

Following this, many others voice their support for Manuel and one of their peers, also in the audience, approaches at the end of the session to talk about how they can support them with meeting people and socialising more with people their own age. Manuel is unsure but agrees to try this. Two months later, Manuel is able to share with his personal advisor at the university that the experience of the Schwartz Round has changed their life; they have gained confidence as they now have a social network outside their family, they feel able to engage and relate to their peers and this has helped them to feel happier in all areas of their life. This has been noted by their line manager who shared feedback on the way they interact with their colleagues in a lighter way, how others have commented how much they enjoy working with Manuel and how their value within the team has increased.

Organisations that are resilient are able therefore to support staff in providing care as the environment reflects those positive approaches needed for resilience to thrive. This in turn can enable individuals to develop strong resilience in the roles they complete and can influence leadership, as Goleman discusses. Therefore, leadership as a nursing associate is something that you may develop as you progress with your own resilience development, supporting the quality of care you deliver to patients or service users throughout your career. Leadership in nursing associate practice is explored in more depth in *Understanding Leadership for Nursing Associates* (Cowls et al., 2023).

Chapter summary

This chapter has identified the importance of personal resilience to manage and maintain healthy relationships. The nature of patients' resilience, and the interaction you have with them, affects the patient experience and your own self-management. Emotions play an important role in how you feel, so being able to recognise and respond to patients when they are experiencing stressors is an important mechanism in maintaining your own caring responsibilities as a SNA/NA. Adaptive and maladaptive coping mechanisms have been explored to highlight strategies to enable developing resilience through mindfulness and laughter. Goleman's emotional intelligence model has been identified as a way of increasing awareness of the components of emotional intelligence to strengthen your relationships with others. The role of organisational resilience, the impact this has on a workforce and the use of Schwartz Rounds to enable stronger resilience have been identified, along with the NMC (2024a) standards that link to resilience, clinical decision-making and subsequent impact on patient care.

Activities: Brief outline answers

Activity 3.1 Reflection (page 37)

You may have recognised how you respond to stressful situations and the strategies you use to enable you to manage these effectively. Sometimes, you may not manage but then you work your way through to overcome the situation to move forward. Your coping strategies will be unique to you and unique to situations as they present themselves; for example, you may feel more resilient in some situations compared to others. Recognising this, and the strategies that help you navigate them, will help you in embedding these strategies in future.

Activity 3.2 Reflection (page 40)

What things do you think you need to be a resilient person both professionally and privately?

The ability to recognise when something is causing you stress or feelings of anxiety. Being able to reflect on uncomfortable feelings or challenges that you face.

Being able to seek support from others.

Being able to take actions that help you feel happier, more relaxed, such as taking a walk or being in the natural environment, doing something creative, spending time with people you care about and who care about you.

Self-care; making sure you eat well and have a good sleep routine.

Activity 3.4 Reflection (page 43)

When you are using your computer, silence email notifications so you are not inter-rupted, make a specific time to read and respond to these. Try to avoid social media when focusing on a project, research has demonstrated that social media not only impacts on your emotional well-being but also reduces focus; so leave your phone in another room when you need to study or complete assignments.

Activity 3.5 Work-based learning (page 44)

Factors that can impact an organisation's resilience include financial pressures, increased demand on services, political change with policy direction, quality assurance measurement through CQC or commitment of staff.

Factors that impact staff resilience include support for continued professional development, leadership approaches, supportive supervision of staff, feeling valued and listened to.

Activity 3.6 Critical thinking (page 45)

Challenges for staff to participate in Schwartz Rounds:

Time – being able to be released from a work environment.

Attitudes towards participation if line manager does not see the benefit.

It can feel daunting as you are sharing your own experiences.

This can make you vulnerable.

Annotated further reading

Watch this video where Goleman discusses: What is emotional intelligence www.youtube.com/watch?v=Y7m9eNoB3NU

To enhance understanding of your own emotional intelligence, read and ask three questions from:

Goleman, D. and Nevarez, M. (2018) 'EMOTIONAL INTELLIGENCE: Boost Your Emotional Intelligence with These 3 Questions', *Harvard Business Review Digital Articles*, pp. 2–5. https://hbr.org/2018/08/boost-your-emotional-intelligence-with-these-3-questions

Watch this Ted Talk Video with Sarah Jayne Blakemore: The mysterious workings of the adolescent brain (2012). This 15-minute video explains executive and social cognition of the adolescent brain that will help you understand why some young adults may not understand, respond or see things in the same way as people further into adult life. http://www.youtube.com/watch?v=6zVS8HIPUng

Role modelling and professional relationships

NMC (2024A) *STANDARDS OF PROFICIENCY FOR NURSING ASSOCIATES*

This chapter will address the following platforms and proficiencies.

Platform 1: Being an accountable professional

1.3 Understand the importance of courage and transparency and apply the Duty of Candour, recognising and reporting any situations, behaviours or errors that could result in poor care outcomes.

1.4 Demonstrate an understanding of, and the ability to challenge or report, discriminatory behaviour.

1.9 Communicate effectively using a range of skills and strategies with colleagues and people at all stages of life and with a range of mental, physical, cognitive and behavioural health challenges.

1.11 Provide, promote, and where appropriate advocate for, non-discriminatory, person-centred and sensitive care at all times. Reflect on people's values and beliefs, diverse backgrounds, cultural characteristics, language requirements, needs and preferences, taking account of any need for adjustments.

1.16 Act as an ambassador for their profession and promote public confidence in health and care services.

Platform 4

4.1 Demonstrate an awareness of the roles, responsibilities and scope of practice of different members of the nursing and interdisciplinary team, and their own role within it.

4.2 Demonstrate an ability to support and motivate other members of the care team and interact confidently with them.

4.5 Demonstrate an ability to prioritise and manage their own workload, and recognise where elements of care can safely be delegated to other colleagues, carers and family members.

4.7 Support, supervise and act as a role model to nursing associate students, healthcare support workers and those new to care roles; review the quality of the care they provide, promoting reflection and providing constructive feedback.

> ## Chapter aims
>
> - Identify the role of your professional relationships in effective team working.
> - Explore role modelling and how this influences the way you work with others.
> - Recognise the links to effective team working and delivery of high-quality patient care.
> - Understand the impact that poor team relationships has on care delivery.
> - Identify the background to the development of the nursing associate in the context of effective teams in health and care services.

Introduction

This chapter will start by exploring beliefs and values you have and the values and behaviours expected of all registrants. The role of coaching and role modelling behaviours will be explored to support deeper understanding for the development of team working within your professional practice and how this supports learning within the care environment. The subsequent impact on the quality of care experienced by patients will be discussed to highlight the roles the Francis Report (2013) and The Shape of Caring Review (Health Education England, 2015) had in influencing the development of the nursing associate role.

The role of resilience in developing and maintaining professional relationships, as discussed in Chapter 3, is key for effective team working. Being able to recognise vulnerability in yourself and your colleagues, and having confidence to raise this, is a professional responsibility of all registrants to support quality patient care. In all health and care settings, you will get a range of personalities, ages and cultures with varying attitudes and behaviours. Being able to understand your own attitudes and behaviours, thinking about the NMC (2018a) *The Code: professional behaviours for nurses, midwives and nursing associates*, will enable you to reflect on the impact they have on team working and patient care.

Assessment of values and behaviours

Values and behaviours underpin assessment for apprentices and the NMC, so it is important to consider your own values and how these affect your behaviours. Values are principles or qualities that are considered valuable or desirable to you as an individual. For example, if you grew up in a close family, you may value family time and be supported by the closeness of your family; although you may be hindered by the demands made by family on your time, you accept this. If your family lived far apart and did not connect very often during your childhood, you may not value family time in the same way. You may be more independent and self-sufficient, but find it harder to manage stressful situations as you have fewer support networks; or you may have developed a wide network of friends that are a support network. Either way, how you connect with people within your family and your friends will influence how you connect with colleagues and patients.

The behaviours you exhibit are the results of your values; therefore, it is important to explore your own beliefs and values to see what is important to you and what influence this has on your working relationships. In Chapter 1, you used a SWOB self-assessment to identify strengths and weaknesses, opportunities and barriers to develop an action plan to manage and overcome deficits. In Chapter 2, you identified how to reflect on your experiences. Both these tools can be used to explore your own values and behaviours to recognise the significance these have on your professionalism and how this influences your professional relationships.

Table 4.1   Values

Acceptance	Achievement	Adventure	Authenticity	Beauty
Ambition	Accountability	Altruism	Being the best	Belonging
Balance	Bravery	Challenge	Clarity	Community
Creativity	Curiosity	Discovery	Diversity	Empathy
Enthusiasm	Ethics	Expertise	Family	Fitness
Career	Collaboration	Commitment	Compassion	Competence
Connection	Contentment	Confidence	Dignity	Environment
Freedom	Friendliness/ Friendship	fulfilment	Fun	Generosity
Efficiency	Equality	Excellence	Fairness	Faith
Financial stability	Forgiveness	Future generations	Giving back	Grace
Harmony	Home	Humility	Honesty	Hope
Gratitude	Grit	Growth	Health	Humour
Independence	Integrity	Intelligence	Intimacy	Kindness
Joy	Leadership	Learning	Loyalty	Mindfulness
Inclusion	Initiative	Intuition	Job security	Justice
Knowledge	Legacy	Leisure	Making a difference	Optimism
Nature	Openness	Passion	Personal growth	Partnership
Order	Parenting	Patience	Patriotism	Peace
Perseverance	Personal fulfilment	Pride	Recognition	Reliability
Playfulness	Popularity	Power	Religion	Resilience
Respect	Romance	Safety	Security	Self-expression
Resourcefulness	Risk-taking	Self-discipline	Self-respect	Serenity
Sportsmanship	Success	Thrift	Time	Tradition
Travel	Trust	Truth	Understanding	Uniqueness

Activity 4.1   Reflection and critical thinking

From the list in Table 4.1, which values do you identify with? Make a list under the heading 'values'. You can add your own if they are not listed. Use Table 4.3 in brief outline answers at the end of the chapter.

Identify the most important things to you in life. Make a list under the heading 'values'.

(Continued)

(Continued)

Why are these important to you?

How does this influence your behaviour? Make a list of these under the heading 'behaviours'.

What impact does this have on others? Add a list next to the behaviours you have identified.

Using your SWOB template from Chapter 1, identify strengths and weaknesses within your values.

Can you identify what opportunities these create for you as a developing nursing associate?

Identify one value that you do not have but think is important for nursing associate practice.

Consider why you have not already got this value and how you can develop and incorporate it into your life.

Identify someone who exhibits this value; what behaviours do you see that shows this value and what do you admire about them?

What barriers are there that may prevent you from developing this? What actions can you take to overcome those barriers?

Now create a SMART action plan, as discussed in Chapter 1, outlining the value, the actions you need to take, how you will measure your success and the time frame you intend to do this in. Make sure you are being specific and realistic.

This activity is a personal reflection, so the outline answer at the end of the chapter provides guidance only.

NHS constitution (Department of Health and Social Care, 2023)

Working within health services is governed by the NHS Constitution, which has the core National Health Service (NHS) values at its heart and strongly links to the 6 Cs.

Working together for patients

Patients should come first and be fully involved in their care decisions. Staff both within the NHS and in other health and care services, family, carers, communities, as well as patients, are considered before the requirements of your organisational boundaries. This relates to Care and Courage from the 6 Cs, for example, through speaking up when you see something that is not right. This is crucial to link to NMC (2024a) *Standards of Proficiency for Nursing Associates* 1.3 and 1.4.

Respect and dignity

The expectation is that you value each individual, patients, carers, families and staff, with respect for their own hopes, needs, things they value, their abilities and limitations. You need to listen to them and understand and respond to them with openness and honesty about what is possible and what is not. This relates to Compassion and Communication within the 6 Cs and links to NMC (2024a) *Standards of Proficiency for Nursing Associates* 1.3 and 1.11.

Commitment to quality of care

The trust that patients and service users place on you has to be earned through getting it right when providing fundamental care that is safe and effective to support a positive care experience. Feedback from service users is crucial in ensuring the care you give meets their needs, which is why the NMC expects all pre-registration nursing associates to gain patient feedback as part of their assessment of practice. It is easy to pick a service user who you had a positive interaction with; however, it is more important to gain feedback from those where you have been challenged as you will learn more from that. This is where reflection is key to exploring how you acted, why you acted that way and how you may need to change your behaviour to support meeting this part of the NHS Constitution. This also aligns with Commitment within the 6 Cs (Cummings, 2012).

Compassion

Compassion involves treating people's needs with humanity and kindness by identifying the things we can do for them that give comfort and alleviates suffering. You can do this by making time for your patients, their families and carers, or your colleagues. You should not wait to be asked but have the capacity to recognise these needs and respond to them. This also links to Compassion within the 6 Cs.

Improving lives

By working to meet your patients' and service users' needs, you are aiming to improve their health and well-being, as well as ensuring a positive experience of NHS services. You will see your own contribution towards making things better for patients, but also supporting improvements within practice to contribute towards healthier communities. Competence and Commitment are important elements of the 6 Cs in achieving this.

Everyone counts

The NHS has limited resources, therefore making these work for the whole community, being inclusive and ensuring people are not discriminated against with a care experience by understanding that sometimes, we need to give more to some than others, through Care and Commitment of the 6 Cs. This aligns to NMC (2024a) *Standards of Proficiency for Nursing Associates* 1.4 and 1.11.

To enable you as a developing health and care professional achieve these, you have to be able to understand your core values and the impact these can have on those you work with and those you care for. The NHS Constitution is updated every five years to reflect changes both within society and the realities of what services can provide, with expectations of the public and staff alike. Working alongside to complement the NHS Constitution, the 6 Cs – care, communication, compassion, courage, commitment, competence – all have a place within the care that you give as shown in the links discussed.

There are a number of organisations that are involved in quality assurance of the NHS and care services and development of values within them. It is important to be aware of these, particularly when your organisation is being inspected by the Care Quality Commission (CQC) as they have their own values (CQC, 2022b) (see annotated reading). The World Health Organization (WHO) also influences the values and skills for those who work within health and care services (see annotated reading).

Activity 4.2   Reflection

Now you have identified your core values, the behaviours you have that show those values and one value you would like to have, reflect on how these relate to the NHS Constitution and the 6 Cs.

This activity is a personal reflection, so the outline answer at the end of the chapter provides guidance only.

Now you have a better understanding of your own core values, you can think about how you are influenced through colleagues and peers, and how you influence others in the practice environment.

Role modelling

Role modelling has been a core part of healthcare practice for many generations, through sharing standards of behaviour to others. This can be shared through articulating expectations but also through actions, although arguably, you need to know and understand the reasoning behind the actions to make sense of this. As nursing is a respected profession, it is a key expectation of the public and NMC alike, that you are morally obliged to behave professionally at all times, in keeping with the NMC (2018a) *The Code* through your individual approach to professionalism. This also supports the NMC (2024a) *Standards of Proficiency for Nursing Associates* 1.16 and 4.7.

Individual professionalism is advocated to be able to share what professionalism looks like through your positive core values and behaviours towards diversity, being supportive to other students and colleagues, celebrating professional success, treating people with positive regard and being able to give meaningful and constructive feedback to others (NMC, 2018b). Although it has many positive influences, the potential is that role modelling can have negative influences as well, as not all healthcare professionals always work within these principles. The impact of this will be explored later in the chapter.

Activity 4.3   Work-based learning

Watch this Ted talk by Larisa Halilović (2021) on core values and your inner compass before completing the reflective activity below.

www.ted.com/talks/larisa_halilovic_core_values_your_inner_compass

Thinking about your own core values, reflect on the behaviours you have observed in others within your placements.

Would you want to be like them, or do you see areas for improvement in their behaviours?

Have you been inspired and have aspirations to be like a nurse, nursing associate or care assistant you have worked with in practice? If so, what was it about their practice that you admired?

Have you observed poor behaviours of any nurses, nursing associates or care assistants? If so, did you feel able to say anything about this to anyone? If not, how can you think about how to do this in future?

Consider the responsibilities you have to speak up and advocate for patients and service users; if it is not acceptable, then they are receiving poor care.

An outline answer is provided at the end of the chapter, but remember that each situation is different, so your experience in clinical practice may differ.

It could be argued that people who enter a healthcare profession do so with the best intentions; however, over time, people can become desensitised to other's needs, the impact of stress within the workplace, or unsupportive management, can all result in challenges to attitudes and behaviours you may witness. It is not unusual to feel helpless when faced with tasks you are not equipped to handle. To enable you to support others through being a role model, you will need to be able to articulate how and why certain behaviours are more effective in meeting patients' needs, as well as working within the parameters, or scope, of your professional practice. There are a number of ways you can work to support this learning; however, coaching has been identified as a supportive approach and will help you meet NMC (2024a) *Standards of Proficiency for Nursing Associates* 1.9, 1.10 and 4.2.

Role modelling therefore involves a range of processes that include observation and emulation of others' behaviour, experimentation and assimilation (as discussed in Chapter 2 with Kolb's learning cycle) to develop general, professional, expertise. Role models are a strong complement to teaching in practice as behaviour is learnt by observing others to give you an idea of what is expected and related to social learning theory developed by Bandura (1977). However, not everything can be learnt and understood through this process alone. When role modelling behaviours need to be further developed to enable others to understand the reasons why you behave in a certain way within practice, you can consider how to share that knowledge through coaching them.

Case study: Fatima

Fatima is a registered Nursing Associate supervising a SNA, Harold, on placement. After the first week, Fatima has noticed that Harold is freezing out other support staff by ignoring them and not including them in the team discussions. These behaviours are creating tension in the wider team, with belittling views on SNAs. Fatima feels they are being seen in the same way, despite being an integrated part of the team prior to this and decides to discuss this with their manager. The manager helps Fatima recognise the underpinning issue and the negative impact this is having on Fatima's health and well-being, and that it is affecting management of patient care. They discuss what attitudes and behaviours they have observed and that an action plan is needed to address them.

Fatima feels uncertain as they have not experienced an issue like this before, so they spend some time reflecting on the behaviours they feel they have displayed since Harold started in the placement. When they meet Harold, they ask what attitudes and behaviours they have observed within the team. Harold identifies a number of positive behaviours that Fatima identified but states that support staff do not know how to behave as they are putting down their contributions when they are working together to deliver patient care. Fatima asks why Harold has not raised this before; Harold states they felt intimidated as this is a close team and felt they would not be believed or supported. Fatima then asks what actions Harold

(Continued)

(Continued)

has taken to try and address the situation for themselves, to which they reply, 'I just ignore them as I know what I am doing is right'.

Fatima asks Harold how they would feel being ignored in that way and Harold suddenly recognises that they would raise this as an issue with Fatima as it is not a positive behaviour. Fatima supports Harold by recognising the behaviour the support staff have shown is not a positive one but that the response Harold has shown is also not a positive one. They ask Harold to complete a reflection on the attitudes and behaviours experienced and to look at the NMC (2018a) The code of behaviours to identify what they could and should have done instead. Together, they create an action plan to demonstrate the professional behaviours that are expected, including apologising to support staff. Harold also recognises that they could address the behaviour displayed towards them in a similar way to Fatima's approach to them.

Activity 4.4 Reflection

Reflect on an experience you have had where someone's behaviour towards you caused you to feel uncomfortable, uncertain or undermined your confidence in practice.

What behavioural response did you display? Did you, like Harold in the case study, respond with equally unhelpful behaviour?

What other behaviours could you have responded with?

How easy is it to address negative behaviours within the team?

This activity is a personal reflection, so the outline answer at the end of the chapter provides guidance only.

In the case study, Fatima used a mixture of approaches to supporting the SNA and resolving the situation, initially reflecting on their own behaviours to consider what behaviours the SNA would have observed and possibly tried to emulate, then used open questions to understand the SNA's experience and for them to recognise the impact and inappropriateness of their behaviour. This is a coaching approach and has been encouraged as a learning and teaching strategy in healthcare environments (Richardson et al., 2023).

Coaching

Central to the ethos of coaching is the idea that within a supportive and trusting relationship, coaches can help you to develop in order to support you to meet your potential. You may recognise this from your own learning experiences. It can be used to enable you to identify what helps and hinders when learning something new, as well as help you start to support others to learn new things.

It can feel a big responsibility to share knowledge – others will want you, and you will want other people to get the right knowledge, develop the clinical skills correctly and demonstrate appropriate professional behaviours. Understanding your own values and behaviours and reflecting on these to pick out important points can help you identify areas you feel more confident in. This is where professionalism is a key consideration.

Professionalism is underpinned in practice through the use of evidence-based decision-making by those who share the same values and had the same education. The role of relationships within this is important as these support closer working relationships, improve productivity and meeting the needs of patients and the service. The impact on those working in the environment is associated with stronger job satisfaction as well. Over time, as you develop your knowledge and skills, you will start supporting others in developing their knowledge and skills, and this is an important step in your professional development. It shows that you are trusted and your knowledge and skills valued, although you may not always feel as confident in your own knowledge and skills as others project.

When you start off supporting others within practice, it can feel quite daunting, although it is not that difficult to transform your knowledge (know-how) into 'know-how-to' for others. It just requires some tools and techniques that you can learn and practise to make it work. We all possess an almost endless list of know-hows that at some point someone might call on us to share. When that happens, it is how prepared will you be to meet the challenge of transforming your know-how into their ability to perform. Coaching is an effective way to approach this.

Understanding theory: GROW model (Whitmore et al., 2013)

The GROW model is one of the best-known models to structure learning. The model breaks a coaching session into four phases: Goals, Reality, Options and Way forward. You may need to identify what the gap is in the person's knowledge through discussion on the situation, before moving on to detailing the preferred outcome or goal and then, through this gap analysis process, developing action steps or strategies to achieve a stated aim.

The different coaching stages can also be thought of as:

1. **Rationale:** Explain why they should learn this and how it applies to their work.
2. **Objectives:** Point out what they need to be able to do.
3. **Activities:** Give them things to do. Make these interesting. Do not bore them.
4. **Evaluation:** Check to see if they have learnt.

The key point here for teaching, is that as a coach you need to have informed flexibility. You need to be comfortable in moving from a highly structured approach to a less structured approach as the situation unfolds. The needs of the learner are the most important consideration, and how the coach can be flexible in meeting the needs of the learner, not how attached the coach is to any specific model. GROW, and other models, are tools to be used, not ideologies to be rigidly adhered to.

To start using this approach, you will need to identify a goal that the learner wants to achieve. If a learner identifies this, then they are more likely to be motivated to achieve this. Having set a goal, the conversation moves on to discussing the reality, what is really happening. This is where you can raise anything you feel needs to be addressed for the learner to be successful if they are unable to reflect and see this for themselves. Frequently, at this stage ideas are uncovered which lead to the goal being refined, therefore, you will need to revisit and help the learner to redefine it. Having redefined the goal, and explored the reality again, you will then consider what options are available until a range of action steps are identified. Sometimes at this point the goal will be revisited again to make sure that the options meet the goal, or alternatively the options may have to be refined. Finally, you can move into the way forward stage and start to help the learner detail specific action steps. It is never clear at the start how the session will actually evolve, and you need to be flexible with how you support your learner (Stolovitch and Keeps, 2021).

Benner novice to expert (1982)

When you first start out trying to accomplish something new, you are a novice as you have never tried or been exposed to the knowledge or skill you are learning. As a SNA, you may have experiences from working in healthcare environments, so therefore you may be a novice in some areas, and an advanced beginner, competent or proficient for other skills depending on your knowledge and experience. Sometimes you may have experience, for example of venepuncture as a practical skill, but lack knowledge on the physiological structure of the cardiovascular system, or why the person is having the blood sample taken. This would mean you are competent in taking the sample but a novice or advanced beginner in the underpinning knowledge on this. Wherever you are in your learning journey, understanding there is a process that enables you to acquire knowledge and skills to move you from a novice to advanced beginner, onto being competent – as assessed through practice assessment documents and academic assessment – to then be able to further refine these to become proficient, and even become expert can support your learning journey. This is not necessarily a process where you have to move through each stage. You may move between stages as you develop towards competency, and competency is not something that is simply achieved and there forever; therefore, reflective practices are necessary to enable continued exploration of experiences, knowledge and skills to recognise when these may require further practice or learning. If you do not use your new knowledge or skills, you may move back to advanced beginner or even novice. Benner's framework (see Table 4.2) will be explored in greater detail in Chapter 7. This is one of the requirements of professionalism, recognising that knowledge and skills need to be maintained, and why the NMC expects revalidation to demonstrate continued learning and competency through continued professional development throughout your career. This will be explored further in Chapter 8.

Table 4.2   Benner stage definitions and strategy examples

Stage	Definition	Potential strategies for skills and knowledge acquisition
Novice	You have no previous experience which makes it difficult to decide what is most relevant to accomplish first.	Teach simple, objective concepts/attributes that are easily identified
Advanced beginner	You have enough real-world experience that you can recognise what is needed when it is related to rules and guidelines.	Increase assistance and support in setting priorities to clients' needs by providing guidelines for recognising patterns
Competent	You have been on the job for some time and are able to see actions in terms of goals or plans and you work in an efficient and organised manner to reach the desired outcome.	Offer in service education or opportunities
Proficient	You perform by using evidence that provides direction to see a situation as a whole.	Use case studies to stimulate critical thinking especially in situations with principles or rules that are contradictory
Expert	You grasp the situation and understand what needs to be accomplished beyond rules, guidelines.	Provide opportunities for experts to share their skills and knowledge and also their analytical abilities to solve new situations

As a novice coach, the uncertainty you may experience can cause anxiety and frustration and as a novice coach, you may react to these feelings by sticking to the model (Stolovitch and Keeps, 2021). Over time, you will develop confidence in using coaching as an approach and will be able to see how you move through Benner's novice to expert framework (Table 4.2).

Case study: Juliana

Juliana has been working within a community nursing team for the last 5 years. They have a range of knowledge and skills around wound care, supporting patients within their own home and working with GPs, physiotherapists and speech and language therapists in the community. The placement allocation is shared and Juliana is allocated an Accident and Emergency placement. Initially, Juliana is excited and is looking forward to the experience; however, as the time draws closer, a SNA working in the department starts to explain what to expect. Juliana suddenly feels they lack the knowledge and skills needed for the placement and worries that the Practice Assessor and Supervisors will think they are not a very good SNA.

On the first day of placement, the Practice Assessor talks to Juliana and asks about her previous experiences. Juliana confides their concerns and together they identify some basic skills and knowledge Juliana needs to acquire to ensure they are safe. For the first 2 days, they are allocated to a healthcare assistant who shows them around the department, explaining the different areas and routines within this. By the end of the second shift, Juliana feels they have a good understanding of routines and has had an opportunity to practise taking basic observations, a skill they do not use in the community regularly, although they are trained in this.

Over the next few weeks, Juliana and the Practice Assessor work together and at the mid-point interview, they identify that Juliana has achieved a competent level of taking observations, recording and is able to demonstrate understanding of what the observations mean, in terms of escalating to the nurse or doctor when a patient is deteriorating.

By the time Juliana has finished the placement, they reflect on this particular skill and recognise that they have moved from novice to competent. Now they have achieved this, Juliana wants to remain competent and returns to the community team with a learning objective of continuing to use skills in taking observations. This is discussed with the team; Juliana's new knowledge and skill in taking observations is recognised and they are asked to run regular skills update sessions for the community nursing team to ensure everyone's knowledge and skills remain current.

Juliana is being a role model to a range of professionals they work with, from healthcare assistant through to managers, as they are able to demonstrate knowledge and skills in a specific area. As a result, they are moving from competent to proficient, as they are able to both demonstrate the practical skill whilst explaining what is occurring physiologically, as well as apply softer skills, such as communication and compassion, in the way the skills are completed with patients. Juliana's knowledge and skills are valued by the team and this helps Juliana feel more confident in their role as a SNA and a valued member of the team.

If a task offers you little challenge to complete well, it should be easy for you to simply 'show someone else how to do it'. It is intuitive, but research has demonstrated that what appears to be simple, whether it is a member of staff providing directions to a visitor, or a fellow worker helping to safely move a patient, things often go wrong, things happen and simple becomes confusing. Both you, the coach, and the learner can become frustrated and you end up asking yourself, if I know so much, why can't they learn?

Once you have several skills and specific knowledge, you could think of this as having the knowledge needed. This entails you being able to get the job done in an expert fashion and demonstrate the skills and knowledge to accomplish what the learner requires. You may think of having the knowledge needed as a highly qualified, recognised expert, but being an expert of a specific subject is not necessary. If you know more than someone who needs to learn, then you possess the necessary knowledge. Imagine that I am lost in a hospital and desperately need to find the toilet. You work in the hospital, have used the toilet many times, and know exactly where the nearest one is. You have the necessary knowledge in getting to the closest toilet. Anyone who has the skills and knowledge to accomplish what the learner requires can share that with others; however, knowing how to do something (or possessing know-how) does not mean that you can effectively communicate your knowledge to another person. Being able to do something and being able to explain, demonstrate, show, or guide how to perform the task are two different things. Expertise is the ability to perform, but not necessarily explain how it is done. Experts and novices think and process information differently; the more you know about the subject, the bigger the gap between you and the learner; therefore, you can get to the toilet with no problem but the question is whether you can you help me get there on my own.

This sharing of your knowledge and skills is the next step in your professional development within your team and will depend on where you are within your learning journey, as you all develop at different rates depending on your past experiences and the learning culture within your placement areas.

Development of the nursing associate role

The culture of the healthcare environment is a crucial part of delivering safe, effective care, but sadly, healthcare cultures can sometimes become unsupportive, with staff working in isolation rather than as a team. There can be challenges with clashes of ideas, values and behaviours that create cultures where you feel unwelcome and unvalued. This is known as a **toxic culture** – one where bullying, defensiveness and hostility rule the care environment with negative effects on staff well-being and potentially this can result in poor patient care. This has been identified and explored by a number of reviews, the most prominent being the Francis Report (Mid Staffordshire NHS Foundation Trust Public Inquiry 2013), which reviewed failings at the Mid-Staffordshire hospital. It highlighted a toxic culture that resulted in failings in patient care and made 290 recommendations to improve these. The NMC (2024a) *Standards of Proficiency for Nursing Associates* linked at the start of the chapter all have links to the outcomes of the report. Following this report, the Cavendish Review (2013) also identified challenges around pre- and post-registration nursing and education of care assistants across health and social care environments. This resulted in the *Shape of Caring Review* (Health Education England, 2015) being jointly commissioned by Health Education England (HEE) and the NMC, which made recommendations for education and training in health and care services. This was to ensure that the services would be able to meet the changing needs of patients, knowledge and medical developments, as more demands would be made on services. The final report, *Raising the Bar* (Health Education England, 2015), amongst other things, emphasised the need to value care assistants and to widen access for them to enter the nursing profession by reducing barriers and encouraging employers to 'grow your own' nursing workforce. This needed to use a 'widening participation' approach as it was recognised that healthcare assistants often did not have the academic entry requirements for completing pre-registration nursing programmes in universities.

One of the recommendations was for HEE to work with universities and employers to develop a standardised work-based learning route. It is from this that the Nursing Associate role was developed by HEE and later supported by the NMC, who agreed to regulate through adding nursing associates to the register. It is the process of registration and meeting the knowledge, skills, values and behaviours required by the NMC that underpin the curriculum you are studying. Professional **identity** is highlighted as being your knowledge, skills and responsibility being developed. How you perceive your identity and how your colleagues responded to your role, have all been seen as being valued by nursing associates, although challenges around the scope of your practice is still an area that requires further refinement (King et al., 2024).

Activity 4.5   Work-based learning

Reflect on how your role has been developed and supported within your main area of practice.

Consider how you have been supported by your team in developing the knowledge and skills through your learning so far.

Has this changed the way you are perceived by the team? If so, how and why do you think that is?

What differences can you see in the way you approach your team with your thoughts and ideas? Have you developed more confidence in speaking up?

Does the team value the nursing associate role, or are there challenges in understanding the scope of your practice?

Consider what is needed to improve any negative perceptions within the team, who and where you can gain support from, and how you can continue to grow within the scope of your role.

This activity is a personal reflection. An outline answer is provided at the end of the chapter, but remember that each situation is different, so your experience in clinical practice is likely to differ.

Barriers created by poor understanding of your role and resistance from others around the development of the nursing associate as a role can be frustrating but it is important to keep your focus on demonstrating the values and behaviours outlined in the NMC (2018a) *The Code* and the NMC (2024a) *Standards of Proficiency for Nursing Associates*. In doing so, you are using role modelling to show your colleagues, students and others within the care environment, that you value the knowledge and skills you are acquiring and have a passion for learning and delivering the highest quality patient care you can. You cannot govern others' thoughts, but you can demonstrate the professionalism that is valued by registrants. Over time, this will enable the nursing associate role to become embedded into nursing practice and recognised for the valuable contribution the role brings to a range of health and care settings.

Overcoming barriers can be challenging, working with your Practice Assessor, Practice Supervisor, Academic Assessor and line manager, as well as making your tutors aware of any challenges you experience, will help address these. This is not an easy thing to do; however, in doing this, you will be demonstrating NMC (2018a) *The Code* 1.3, the Duty of Candour, where you have an obligation to raise any concerns about the potential risk of poor outcomes or experiences for patients and service users, as potentially, if you are unsupported, this may impact on the quality of care you are able to provide.

Chapter summary

This chapter started by identification of your own values and behaviours to enable you to understand the things that are important to you and how these can influence how others work and respond to you. The requirements of the NHS Constitution were highlighted and links made between this, the 6 Cs and your own values was developed to embed this within your practice. By doing this, you have considered how role modelling works to demonstrate the knowledge and skills valued within the profession and the link this has with professionalism. The role of coaching as a way of developing knowledge and skills has been introduced to explore positive ways of sharing your knowledge and skills with others. This was then discussed in terms of challenges with healthcare culture, where toxic cultures have resulted in poor patient care, with subsequent reports and reviews resulting in changes to the education and development of care assistants across health and social care. These changes enabled your role as a SNA to be developed, although it is recognised as a new role, there are still barriers to this within practice. You have seen how you can continue to promote professional values and behaviours through the way you manage yourself, recognising the barriers and considering ways to overcome these through continued role modelling of those values and behaviours. The links between this and the requirements of the Duty of Candour will be further expanded on through the role of accountability in Chapter 5.

Activities: Brief outline answers

Activity 4.1 Reflection and critical thinking (page 51)

From the list in Table 4.1, the values identified in Table 4.3 and the responses to questions are examples.

Identify the most important things to you in life.

Table 4.3   Examples of the impact of values and behaviours in practice

Value	Behaviour	Impact
Authenticity	*Genuine interest in people and what is going on around me.*	*People feel able to talk to me.*
Curiosity	*Ask lots of questions.*	*People see I am interested in learning and give me as much time and support as they can, although some people find it irritating so I have to recognise when asking questions is not appropriate.*
Reliability	*Always aim to respond as I have said I would; turn up ready to work; communicate if I am finding something challenging to fulfil.*	*People know they can count on me if they ask me to do something, that I will be there when I need to be.*

Why are these important to you? *Being authentic is important to me as I see when some people are false, those around them feel uncertain and do not trust them.*

How does this influence your behaviour? *I try to be authentic; if I feel uncertain about something, I may be quiet so I do not give the wrong impression.*

What impact does this have on others? *I feel people know they can trust me.*

Using your SWOB template from Chapter 1, identify strengths and weaknesses within your values. You can identify what opportunities these create for you as a developing nursing associate. *Strengths: Honesty, integrity. Weaknesses: I lack knowledge within practice. Opportunities: I can ask for additional guidance on where I need to focus learning.*

Next, identify one value that you do not have but think is important for nursing associate practice. *I would like to have knowledge so that I can feel confident in what I am doing in practice.*

Consider why you have not already got this value and how you can develop and incorporate it into your life. *I have not got knowledge for practice as I have not had much time as a student nursing associate. When I was a HCA I was shown how to do things but not why; I see that I need to know why, so when I qualify, I can make clinical decisions that are safe.*

Identify someone who exhibits this value; what behaviours do you see that shows this value and what do you admire about them? *My Practice Supervisor is a newly qualified nursing associate and they have taught me lots of things I need to know. They are helpful and patient with me, checking that I understand and then coming back every now and then to see that I still remember. This has helped me feel more confident in my new knowledge.*

What barriers are there that may prevent you from developing this? *I do not always understand some of the information I get in learning.*

What actions can you take to overcome those barriers? *I need to go back over my notes and lectures so I can process this. I can also talk to my practice supervisor to help me understand what this means when I am at work.*

Now create a SMART action plan outlining the value, the actions you need to take, how you will measure your success and the time frame you intend to do this in. Make sure you are being specific and realistic.

S = Identify one new thing each week to learn about. M = At the end of each week, my practice supervisor is going to ask me to explain what I have learnt. A = I have to think about small things so I have time to understand it properly; if it is too big, I can break it down into 2 things over 2 weeks. R = I think it is realistic to learn one new thing each week but if we are really busy, I may need to spend more time after work to go through this again. T = This is a weekly plan.

Activity 4.2 Reflection (page 54)

Now you have identified your core values, the behaviours you have that show those values and one value you would like to have, reflect on how these relate to the NHS Constitution and the 6 Cs. *I need to have knowledge to make safe and effective clinical decisions to demonstrate my competence. I need to have good communication to get that knowledge and share my clinical decisions.*

Activity 4.3 Work-based learning (page 54)

Reflect on the behaviours you have observed in others within your placements.

Would you want to be like them, or do you see areas for improvement in their behaviours? I have seen some good attitudes and behaviours from lots of nurses but sometimes, they can get stressed and short when they speak to others. This has made me feel a burden at times, which makes me feel less confident. I understand it is hard for them but if I feel stressed, I try to make sure that I do not talk to people in that way.

Have you been inspired and have aspirations to be like a nurse, nursing associate or care assistant you have worked with in practice? If so, what was it about their practice that you admired? I admire my practice supervisor as they have shown me lots of new things. They are always patient and kind to me, even when I do not understand something. They are kind to patients too.

Have you observed poor behaviours of any nurses, nursing associates or care assistants? If so, did you feel able to say anything about this to anyone? I haven't been able to say anything to the nurses when they are short with me.

If not, how can you think about how to do this in future? I have talked to my practice supervisor about how I feel sometimes; they have said they will help me when I experience this to raise this with the nurse in a professional way.

Consider the responsibilities you have to speak up and advocate for patients and service users; if it is not acceptable, then they are receiving poor care. I feel it is really important to speak up for patients; it is more about speaking up for myself that I struggle with.

Activity 4.4 Reflection (page 56)

Reflect on an experience you have had where someone's behaviour towards you caused you to feel uncomfortable, uncertain or undermined your confidence in practice.

What behavioural response did you display? Did you, like the SNA in the case study respond with equally unhelpful behaviour? *I go quiet when I feel uncomfortable.*

What other behaviours could you have responded with? *I could check with them to see if they are alright before letting them know that they are making me feel undermined.*

How easy is it to address negative behaviours within the team? *I think it is very hard to address negative behaviours in the team; we all have good and bad days and I worry if I say something then I will not be supported in the same way.*

Activity 4.5 Work-based learning (page 61)

Reflect on how your role has been developed and supported within your main area of practice. *I have started to understand why we do certain procedures; I like thinking about anatomy and physiology and how the body works and the way in which disease changes this, as well as how treatments help improve or 'fix' the problem.*

Consider how you have been supported by your team in developing the knowledge and skills through your learning so far. *The team is often very busy but my practice supervisor has been really supportive. I would like to spend more time with the nurses and other members of the team to try and learn from them too.*

Has this changed the way you are perceived by the team? If so, how and why do you think that is? *I think the team works well together; now I have time to understand more about working together. I can see that perhaps I can do more in my role as I gain new knowledge and skills so that others can see how willing I am to learn and be a supportive team member.*

What differences can you see in the way you approach your team with your thoughts and ideas; have you developed more confidence is speaking up? *I can see how I can change the way I approach the team to make them aware of how I feel and the impact this has on my confidence. I haven't done anything about this yet but my practice supervisor is going to help me.*

Does the team value the nursing associate role, or are there challenges in understanding the scope of your practice? *I think the team values my practice supervisor as they rely on them for lots of things that they do not ask me to get involved in. I am not sure they fully understand the role of the SNA, they do not always remember what the registered nursing associate cannot do. This means they have to speak up, which is something I am going to have to work on.*

Consider what is needed to improve any negative perceptions within the team, who and where can you gain support from, and how you can continue to grow within the scope of your role. *My practice supervisor is very confident at speaking up when they are asked to do something that is not within their role. I think that having more than one voice will help them as well as helping me.*

Annotated further reading

Video – GROW model /www.youtube.com/watch?v=_TMM0lhukBg

This video explores the GROW model of coaching to support your understanding of how you can use this within your own practice in supporting others.

Grant, A. M. (2011) 'Is it time to REGROW the GROW model? Issues related to teaching coaching session structures', *Coaching Psychologist*, 7(2), pp. 118–126.

This article will enable you to consider the use of the GROW model, to enhance your critical analysis of information.

Care Quality Commission (CQC) (2022b) Link to values page www.cqc.org.uk/about-us/our-purpose-role/who-we-are

Understanding the role of the CQC will enable you to develop confidence that your values and behaviours meet those required by the CQC to demonstrate the quality of care you deliver to your patients or service users.

World Health Organization (WHO) This web page identifies values and skills for health: www.who.int/about/values

Exploring the values the WHO identify can support critical consideration of your own organisations values. Identifying the similarities and differences between these, questioning whether your organisation is explicit in expressing and implementing these values or whether they are implied can help you develop a strong sense of what values are considered in the wider, global context of health and care services.

Health Education England (2015) Raising the Bar: Shape of Caring: A review of the Future Education and Training of Registered Nurses and Care Assistants. Available at: www.hee.nhs.uk/sites/default/files/documents/2348-Shape-of-caring-review-FINAL.pdf

Reading the recommendations for Theme 4 will strengthen your understanding of the way the review informed the development of the nursing associate role.

Chapter 5

Accountability in nursing associate practice

NMC (2024A) *STANDARDS OF PROFICIENCY FOR NURSING ASSOCIATES*

This chapter will address the following platforms and proficiencies.

Platform 1: Being an accountable professional

1.1 Understand and act in accordance with The Code: Professional standards of practice and behaviour for nurses, midwives and nursing associates, and fulfil all registration requirements.

1.2 Understand and apply relevant legal, regulatory and governance requirements, policies, and ethical frame works, including any mandatory reporting duties, to all areas of practice.

1.3 Understand the importance of courage and transparency and apply the Duty of Candour, recognising and reporting any situations, behaviours or errors that could result in poor care outcomes.

Platform 4: Working in teams

4.1 Demonstrate an awareness of the roles, responsibilities and scope of practice of different members of the nursing and interdisciplinary team, and their own role within it.

4.7 Support, supervise and act as a role model to nursing associate students, healthcare support workers and those new to care roles; review the quality of the care they provide, promoting reflection and providing constructive feedback.

5.6 Understand and act in line with local and national organisational frameworks, legislation and regulations to report risks, and implement actions as instructed, following up and escalating as required.

Chapter aims

- Explore the NMC *Standards of Proficiency for Nursing Associates* for safe and effective practice.
- Understand the role of NMC Code of professional behaviours for nurses, midwives and nursing associates in developing and maintaining professionalism.

(Continued)

(Continued)

- Gain insight into the role of the NMC Standards of student support, supervision and assessment in maintaining safe practice.
- Understand how these standards link to the Duty of Candour, the role of freedom to speak up champions and whistle-blowing.
- Consider the boundaries and scope of practice of the nursing associate role and how these are evolving.

Introduction

The NMC is the regulator for all registrants, whether nurses, midwives or nursing associates. Legally, they have this responsibility as part of the Nursing and Midwifery Order 2001, known as the 'Order', which the government introduced to ensure patient safety and minimum standards of care within care environments. Therefore, all registrants are governed through this legal framework, which requires them to adhere to a range of standards identified by the NMC. The NMC itself has been criticised for poor culture within the organisation, resulting in consultation, an apology and changes within leadership to address these. For registrants to be able to be held accountable, it is argued, the organisation also needs to be held accountable. The current *Standards of Proficiency for Nursing Associates* were developed in 2018 to reflect some changes within care environments and recently updated (NMC, 2024a) to outline role expectations and increasing needs and demands on healthcare professionals across health and care services. The standards were not created to be used in isolation, therefore this chapter explores these in the context of each other.

This chapter explores each of the standards in relation to each other so that you can understand the scope of your responsibilities, and as a registrant, your **accountability**. You will start by exploring the difference between responsibility and accountability before looking at the standards of proficiency, and how this intersects with *The Code* and the role of supervision (NMC, 2018a, 2024c). As a learner on an NMC programme, you are required to have a practice supervisor/practice assessor and academic assessor. On qualifying you will be classed as 'practice supervisor ready' and will therefore be expected to undertake this role with both NA students and nursing students. Therefore, as a learner it is important to develop the knowledge, skills and behaviours as part of your development to be able to carry out this responsibility safely, as you will be accountable for the actions of others under your supervision. While you are learning, your practice supervisor or any registered nurse who delegates a task to you are accountable for this decision; however, you are **responsible** for your actions or omissions in completing the task. It is imperative therefore that you make them aware of the limitations of your knowledge, skills and competencies; this is your responsibility. Any decisions you make in completing a delegated task you have identified you are competent to complete, you then become accountable for your actions or omissions within both the education provider, and the law (Delves-Yates, 2022).

The chapter will then consider how you manage your role, maintain role boundaries and how these may evolve over time, to show how the role of speaking up in practice is necessary. Your responsibilities within the Duty of Candour are explored and the role of freedom to speak up champions and whistle-blowing principles.

Accountability and responsibility

Activity 5.1   Watch

Watch this video for the NMC www.youtube.com/watch?v=iMaVr1M-slA

There is no outline answer at the end of the chapter.

Activity 5.2   Reflection

Reflect on the video to consider how your responsibilities, and accountability for your actions, may change over the duration of your learning.

How will this change when you move into qualified nursing associate practice?

This activity is a personal reflection, so there is no outline answer at the end of the chapter.

Case study: Lulu

Lulu is a second year SNA working within a community mental health team. They have been asked to support a new support worker, Tim, joining the team with becoming familiar with the case load, assessment of service users and related documentation. Lulu is unsure that they should be completing assessment of service users but agrees to take the person under their wing for the first 2 weeks. The first few days are spent explaining what the team does, who has responsibility for what and how they work together to support each other through team reflections each week. They introduce the online documentation system, outlining the different levels of access for different roles with greater responsibilities, as well as stressing the importance of completing the Trust training before accessing the system. Towards the end of the first week, Lulu takes Tim out on their visits, explaining the role they have as an SNA and how they expect this to evolve once qualified and registered with the NMC. Lulu is an experienced practitioner, prior to the SNA programme, they worked in community mental health services for several years. They outline the role Tim will be completing, stressing the need to report any changes to the team leader at the earliest time. During the conversation, Lulu starts to explain about assessment of service users but feels uncomfortable, as although they know the process, it is not within their remit. Lulu decides to explain the process in the context of who holds responsibility and reports back to the team leader on return that they were uncomfortable explaining something they do not complete, as they may not have given the full context, or able to explain why a certain assessment may be used over another. The team leader thanks Lulu for raising their concerns and suggests that Tim should accompany a registered nurse for this.

All registrants are accountable to the NMC for the decisions they make in practice, including **delegation** of tasks to others within the care team. The case study demonstrates that Lulu was able to recognise and raise concerns about the scope of their role. This ensured Tim was able to have a full understanding of the context that different members of the team hold. As a learner, you are not accountable to the NMC; however, you are responsible for ensuring the registered nurse is aware of whether you are competent to complete the delegated task or not. This may be through their assessment of you; however, you also need to state if you feel you are not yet competent, as Lulu did in the case study. You may think accountability and responsibility are the same thing, but within practice there is a significant difference. Being responsible means you act within the scope of your role and competence within the knowledge, skills and experience you have both prior to your training and within this. You may not be able to complete clinical skills you are trained to complete as a healthcare assistant/care assistant/support worker as these are specific to that role, although if you are an apprentice, your employer may have specific policies in place for you to continue with these. It is important that you are clear what you can and cannot complete once you commence your learning in practice, particularly within an external placement. You have responsibility to ensure you work within these boundaries.

Case study: Julie

Julie is a second year SNA who usually works within a mental health environment but is currently on an external placement in a hospital ward. This is their first hospital experience and have no idea of the normal routines. On their first day, they are asked to work in a bay with two healthcare assistants, helping patients with personal care, turning bedbound patients and getting the remainder of patients up into a chair by the bed. Julie has never seen or used the equipment used to move patients before.

Activity 5.3   Critical thinking

What responsibility does Julie have in this situation?

What responsibility does the nurse have?

Who is accountable if Julie uses the equipment incorrectly?

An outline answer is provided at the end of the chapter.

Responsibility involves managing tasks, while accountability focuses on the consequences and ownership of actions, typically involving a single individual. In both case studies, the SNA could have managed the tasks delegated to them, however, as they lacked the necessary knowledge or skills to complete the tasks they were not accountable as they made the nurse aware they lacked that knowledge or skill. This is therefore taking responsibility for their actions and is the founding principle involved with *The Code*.

NMC (2018a) The Code: Professional behaviour for nurses, midwives and nursing associates

The underpinning principles of *The Code* is that it is illegal to practise, or even claim that you are a nurse, midwife of nursing associate if you are not on the register, therefore during your training, you must refer to yourself as a student nursing associate (SNA) or an apprentice nursing associate (ANA), depending on the local agreement. The element of *The Code* that included nursing associates was updated in 2018 from the original publication in 2015 and is currently being reviewed by the NMC (2025). It is part of *The Code* that all registrants use the current version, which is available on the NMC website.

As a legal requirement, *The Code* is not discretionary or negotiable; you are expected to work within this at all times. This includes outside of your professional role, for example on social media, where there is additional guidance on the expectations of your conduct, with the expectation this is read in conjunction with *The Code* and guidance (NMC, 2019b) (see annotated reading) or policies provided by your employer or education provider. Within *The Code*, the NMC has used the term 'nursing' to apply to all those in the 'nursing family', including nursing associates. This is underpinned by the principle of working within your competence, which is the founding requirement for patient safety, with the expectation that those on the register will also promote safe and effective practice. Challenges around this occur when registrants feel unable to speak up about poor practice they witness, poor attitudes and behaviours towards others in the care team or patients. This will be explored further on in this chapter but draws on some of the learning from Chapter 4.

NMC (2024a) *Standards of proficiency for nursing associates*

By now, you will be familiar with the extent of the standards that you have to meet as part of your completion of the nursing associate programme. These were developed following the Health Education England curriculum when the scope of the nursing associate role was taken to the NMC for inclusion in the register, and as a result, the standards were developed in 2018, and redesigned in 2024. This is to ensure that wherever you complete your learning, nursing associates in different parts of the country all have a particular knowledge base. This is achieved through the NMC approving the programmes of study for each individual training provider and all education providers need to follow the NMC *Standards for education and training: Part 3: Standards for pre-registration nursing associate programmes* (NMC, 2024c). As you can see, there are lots of different standards that all need to work together. Sometimes, this can be difficult to process, but if you cannot meet one standard, it is unlikely you are meeting others. The NMC (2024a) *Standards of Proficiency for Nursing Associates* require you to meet the standards set out in *The Code* (NMC, 2018a). This is because the proficiencies require the knowledge, skills and behaviours you need for safe, effective practice and are a legal requirement for Article 15(1) of the Order 2001. The standards are to enable you to understand the scope of your role, and if read alongside the *Standards of Proficiency for Registered Nurses* (NMC, 2024b), you can see how the two roles differ. Within your standard, the main purpose of platform 1 is to ensure these proficiencies are applied to all the other platforms (2–6), so even as individual proficiencies, you need to be able to demonstrate platform 1 alongside. Additionally, the assessment of practice also requires the assessment of professional values throughout your placements, which links to the NMC (2018a) *The Code* pillars: Prioritise people, Practise effectively, Preserve safety and Promote professionalism and trust.

Activity 5.4   Critical thinking

Read the standards of proficiency for registered nurses and nursing associates alongside each other.

How do you think these differ?

In your area of practice, what actions or activities do you think could be considered that of the registered nurse and that of the registered nursing associate?

An outline answer is provided at the end of the chapter, but remember that each situation is different, so your experience in clinical practice may differ.

The responsibility of knowing what you can do as an SNA or registered nursing associate does not fall to you alone; it is also the responsibility of your employer who should define the scope of your role through your job description based on what you achieve through meeting the standards of proficiency. The key difference between the nursing associate and nurse roles includes the scope of practice across the four fields; adult, child, learning disability and mental health, whereas nurses are required to qualify in one field and cannot work across other areas. This gives you unique opportunities to gain knowledge and skills across different environments, for your continued professional development through opportunity to specialise in a given area before continuing education to become a registered nurse within a given field.

NMC (2024c) Standards for student supervision and assessment

Originally published in 2018, these standards were updated in 2023 following updates to standards for education and training, and are split into three parts. Part 1 is the standard for education programmes for nursing and midwifery. Part 2 is the standards that practice assessors and academic assessors are required to adhere to. Part 3 has individual standards for each NMC registered programme, outlining the requirements for each. Similar to *The Code*, these standards were compiled under the legal obligations of 15(1) of the *Order 2001*. These not only ensure you are supported to meet the other standards throughout your education both in practice and in training, but they are also there to protect you and the learning opportunities you have to ensure safe, effective learning for delivering safe and effective patient care. How you are supervised, or supervise other learners will depend on the programme of study and requirements. Part 2 is outlined through three sections: effective practice learning; supervision of students; and assessment of students and confirmation of proficiency. This is the part that you will need to ensure you are familiar with before you start supervising students within practice. This should be completed alongside the Part 3 for the relevant programme – either *Standards of Proficiency Nursing Associates* or *Standards of Proficiency for Registered Nurses* (NMC, 2024c).

Effective learning in practice

The responsibility for learning within practice is supported by further regulations, where the NMC expect approved education institutions (**AEI**), referred to in this book as your education provider, to work with employers to meet the standard frameworks for nursing and midwifery education. This involves joint working to create and provide academic support and overview for positive learning environments. This means that all areas that offer student placements will have a regular audit of the placement that checks there is sufficient support and learning opportunities for nursing students, including nursing associates. To support this, usually the education provider has links with placement areas to support students. This also requires nominated individuals to take responsibility for your learning and assessment, your practice assessor, so that learning supports specific standards of proficiency. This is achieved through the use of Practice Assessment Document (PAD) and your Ongoing Achievement Record (OAR). These documents are a vital record and evidence of your learning, providing an opportunity for your practice supervisors, practice assessor and academic assessor to co-ordinate and communicate with each other to ensure the standards are being met. Additionally, ensuring that you know who and how you can access support to empower you to take responsibility for your learning and support your learning needs. This may include support for a range of diverse needs, such as SpLD (specific learning differences), or accommodating health needs where an occupational health assessment has been completed, as discussed in Chapter 1. This information is private and confidential to you, so your education provider will not share this with placements – this is your responsibility.

It is important to remember that you learn not just from registered nurses or nursing associates – being part of an interprofessional team, you need to know and understand the range of roles, as well as patient experiences, as these help form your overall knowledge and understanding of practice, of being a professional and working within the wider interprofessional team. This is why it is important to identify your own learning needs based on the gaps in your knowledge and experience, and that as a registrant, the needs of your students are supported and that you work within the NMC (2018a) *The Code*.

Activity 5.5   Reflection

Think about the learning you have received so far through your education provider. Review the proficiencies you have already achieved within your practice assessment document (PAD) to see whether you can apply this learning to them.

Where you cannot apply your knowledge, reflect on how having knowledge may enhance your competency.

Using your PAD, review your proficiency assessments to see what clinical skills you still need to achieve.

Identify how and where you could gain exposure to these experiences.

Using the SMART principles from Chapter 1, create learning objectives that you can take to your practice supervisor or assessor so they can support you with accessing the relevant opportunities needed.

This activity is a personal reflection, so there is no outline answer at the end of the chapter.

Once you have identified your learning needs, you can utilise these to enable a proactive approach to your learning in practice. This will demonstrate not only your engagement with learning but support meeting the NMC (2024a) *Standards of Proficiency for Nursing Associates*, work to meeting the requirements of *The Code* (NMC, 2018a), and demonstrate professional values in practice.

Supervision of students

As discussed in Chapter 4, positive role models within practice are a key supportive learning mechanism. During all placements, you should be supervised; however, what that supervision looks like will depend on your level of knowledge and ability as assessed by your practice assessor and supervisor. This is to ensure that you are practising safely and effectively throughout the placement experience. There will be times when this may be difficult, for example, when an assessor or supervisor is unwell, or is needed elsewhere; however, you should always have a practice supervisor available to support you, whether you are facilitated to learn or undertaking learning independently. All registrants can supervise learning, as can other registrants from other professions within health and care services, as long as they understand the NMC (2018a) *The Code* and the scope of your role and have completed relevant supervisor training.

Supervisors must possess the knowledge and skills required for the area they are providing support, and should be supported in this role. They must be able to provide you with constructive feedback for you to develop your practice whilst remaining within the scope of their own practice. They are able to contribute to your assessments through liaising with your practice assessor, and are able to document within your PAD and OAR where a practice supervisor is identified, but not where a practice assessor is identified. They may raise concerns about your practice if they observe actions or behaviours that do not meet the NMC (2018a) *The Code* or *Standards of Proficiency for Nursing Associates* (NMC, 2024a). They are prepared for this role through ensuring they are able to undertake this role and are supported in this. As a newly registered nursing associate, you may be required to supervise others within practice; to help you prepare for this additional responsibility, there are learning opportunities available online or through your local education provider (see annotated reading). If you supervise a student from a programme other than the nursing associate, you will be required to know the standards for that programme to be able to offer the right support.

Activity 5.6   Work-based learning

Think about your own experiences of learning so far. What has been the most helpful learning experience and which has been the least helpful?

What made these helpful or unhelpful?

What would have made a difference to make your learning a more positive experience? What actions can you take to address this?

How can you use this experience when you are required to supervise and support a learner in your practice area?

An outline answer is provided at the end of the chapter, but remember that each situation is different, so your experience in clinical practice is likely to differ.

Assessment of students and confirmation of proficiency

Practice assessors are required to confirm your achievement within clinical settings that demonstrates completion of proficiencies and assessments within your PAD. These are informed and supported through liaison with practice supervisors who have worked to support you throughout your placements; but practice assessors are not able to be both practice supervisor and practice assessor for you; these need to be different people. They also utilise your reflections to review how you assess your own development; the role of reflection on your learning is an important piece of the assessment jigsaw – it is worth remembering that strong reflective practice not only demonstrates your knowledge and skills for practice, but also reflects your attitudes and behaviour towards learning, which also contribute to demonstration of the NMC (2018a) *The Code*. Collaboration between the practice assessor and academic assessor is important to ensure that the learning you have achieved in practice reflects the theory learning you have completed, to enable you to demonstrate application of theory in practice. How your academic and practice assessors communicate may differ at local levels, however, you will have a meeting where all parties come together to discuss and confirm your ability to progress either to year 2, or onto the NMC register and to comply with apprenticeship requirements.

Although assessment of your practice is completed by your practice assessor and your academic assessor, to ensure impartiality, your academic assessor must be a different person for year one and year two of your training. Both academic and practice assessors must have appropriate knowledge and support to enable them to complete this role. Once you qualify, you will be able to undertake both the role of practice assessor and practice supervisor, although some employers may require you to undertake further learning to become an assessor. You can assess those up to and below the level of your training, for example, an SNA or 1st or 2nd year pre-registration nursing student; however, you are unable to assess 3rd year pre-registration nursing students. As an SNA, you can support learning for those up to and below the point of your learning but are unable to assess.

Activity 5.7   Reflection

Reflect on the learning opportunities you have experienced so far to identify both positive and negative experience. You could use the NMC reflection template to start to become familiar with this: www.nmc.org.uk/revalidation/resources/forms-and-templates/.

Identify the barriers to your learning experience and whether anything could be done to overcome these.

Think about what you could do differently to gain different experiences.

Now consider when you have or need to supervise others; this may be a new member of the team or another learner.

Think about your own learning experiences and what made them positive or negative; what can you do to make your learner feel welcome, safe and valued within the care environment?

This activity is a personal reflection, so the outline answer at the end of the chapter provides guidance only.

Supernumerary and protected learning time

As an SNA, you will experience supernumerary placement – these are when you are not counted in the staff numbers and these are crucial learning opportunities for you. If you are an apprentice, in addition to off the job learning away from your usual workplace, you will experience 'protected learning time' within your workplace (see annotated reading), which can be supernumerary; however, this is not an NMC requirement (NMC, 2024c). Protected learning time is time set aside within your normal workload for you to learn new things. This may involve you completing tasks that you completed as part of your previous role; however, you need to start thinking about the learning you get in class and how that applies to these daily routines and tasks. As your knowledge and skills increase, the responsibilities and activities you can complete will be developed within the scope of your practice. As the nursing associate role is relatively new, these may change over time; however, principles around specific competency achievement must be followed to ensure you remain accountable for these.

Case study: Charlie

Charlie has been on the SNA apprenticeship for four months and is starting to feel frustrated. Due to staffing shortages, the time they spend directly with their practice supervisor has been limited and they feel like they are not learning anything new as the tasks they are set are the same as when they were an HCA. Charlie discusses this with the tutor from the training provider who asks whether they have changed anything they do as a result of the learning they have had in university. Charlie identifies that they are more aware of communication with the patients, particularly while completing personal care, they feel they are more person-centred as they are asking and encouraging the patient to do as much for themselves as they can. The tutor asks whether Charlie has reflected on this at all, which they state they have not, so the tutor suggests thinking about each interaction with a patient during these tasks and what they are doing differently, why they are doing it differently and what new knowledge they are using as this is protected learning time.

In the case study you can see that Charlie is not necessarily learning new tasks but learning how to apply new knowledge gained through their studies. Learning comes in different forms: it can be new tasks; it can be reflection on tasks you know how to do, but now you know why they are done the way they are. Another way of identifying both supernumerary and protected learning is to use your initial, mid-point and end of placement interviews to identify what you need to enable you to complete your role when you are a registrant. This will mean managers having a job description for you to work towards. Alternatively, particularly during external placements, you can use the proficiencies to target the areas of practice you still need to achieve, as explored in Activity 5.5.

Scope of practice

The nursing associate role has not been without its critics; initially, some registrants felt it would be 'nursing on the cheap', which would undermine the value of registration (Harold, 2016; Hedayioglu et al., 2023). Others saw it as an opportunity for employers to 'grow their own' nurses as it offered an opportunity for progression onto a pre-registered nursing programme (King et al., 2024). Those you work with both in practice and on placement may take an approach that reflects which point of view they had, and may still have; therefore, you are an advocate for the role and any developments that may evolve over the coming years.

Understanding where the role of the nursing associate came from is an important starting point in changing the hearts and minds of those who may still see this role in a negative way.

The Francis Report (Mid Staffordshire NHS Foundation Trust Public Inquiry 2013) was the first major recognition that there were failings in practice that resulted in poor patient care and abuse. It is likely that your motivations were altruistic when you entered the healthcare environment; you want to make a positive difference to help people who are unwell or unable to meet their own care needs, for whatever reason. Francis identified that the systems and processes were not in place to enable registered professionals to report and follow up on concerns they had; patients, their family and carers lacked the opportunity to report; and reporting was either over complex or not listened to. This resulted in a number of changes, with the development of the 6 C's, and with many organisations updating their values, which you will recognise as the 'vision' or beliefs and values each organisation sets out. As a result, regulators, such as the NMC and GMC produced new standards and guidance, but most importantly, a statutory requirement for a Duty of Candour was identified.

Understanding theory: Duty of Candour (Care Quality Commission, 2022a) and freedom to speak up (NHS England, 2022a)

There are two types of Duty of Candour: statutory and professional.

Statutory

The Care Quality Commission's (CQC, 2022a) Regulation 20 Duty of Candour sets out the requirements for health and social care providers across the UK. This regulation intends to ensure that providers are open and transparent with people who use services and other 'relevant persons' (people acting lawfully on their behalf) about care and treatment.

Professional

The professional Duty of Candour refers to openness and honesty when things go wrong within health and social care services. It is a professional responsibility to be honest with patients when things go wrong. As a doctor, nurse or midwife, allied health professional or health and social care support worker, it is imperative to be open and honest with your patients/service users, colleagues, and employers.

Both the statutory Duty of Candour and professional Duty of Candour have similar aims – to make sure that those providing care are open and transparent with the people using their services, whether or not something has gone wrong.

The development of the Duty of Candour led to the NMC and GMC to develop guidance, which they completed together so all registrants take responsibility for being open and honest with patients, and the organisation, when things go wrong in a healthcare environment, which links to Duty 14 of *The Code* (NMC, 2018a) (see annotated reading). This process looks not only at situations where something has gone wrong and led to harm but where something has gone wrong that could have led to harm. This requires you to share with the patient, their family or carers, when appropriate, when something has gone wrong with the care provided. This must include information on what went wrong, and if known, why, the impact this may have on the patient both in the short and long term, an apology and solution to put things right if that is possible. This will also involve being open and honest with those in the care team, with the issue reported through near miss processes, participating in any investigations or reviews, and if necessary, informing the healthcare regulator Care Quality Commission. This can be challenging within hierarchical environments; you may lack the confidence to speak up, but it is important to recognise that you should encourage people to speak up and not try to hide or evade the issue through excuses or minimisation. Although the guidance is for taking individual responsibility, the NMC does not expect each person within the team involved in an incident to report on behalf of the multi-disciplinary team (MDT) but to ensure that someone reports the incident. As part of the NHS People Promise, NHS England (2022b) (see annotated reading) Freedom to speak up policy, also referred to as whistle-blowing, provides the minimum standards for local policies for speaking up in primary and secondary care and within Integrated Care Boards (ICB). These requirements are aimed at ensuring that you, and all others who work in the NHS and care services, know how to speak up and what happens when you do. Speaking up differs from the Duty of Candour in creating a space for all staff in care services to raise anything that does not feel right. This could include when a process is not working or being followed correctly, you feel discriminated against, or the actions of others are impacting your, your patients' or other colleagues' well-being. One of the challenges that has been raised within the NHS is discrimination; NHS England (2023) have produced a plan that outlines actions intended to develop equality, diversity and inclusion within the NHS based on the protected characteristics embedded within the Equality Act 2010. Some of these experiences may be dealt with through other policies or processes, for example, patient safety or Human Resources processes, but if this is not addressed, you have this additional process available to support you, including accessing your freedom to speak up guardian. If you feel that this is a process you need to follow, you should access information, advice and support from your trade union.

Activity 5.8   Reflection

Reflect on your experiences of poor practice you have observed, whether these are small or serious.

Think about what you did about this, if anything.

What the challenges were for you?

Did the outcomes reflect what you expected from a concern being raised?

This activity is a personal reflection, so there is no outline answer at the end of the chapter.

Case study: George

George settled in the UK from the Philippines seven years ago. They have been a SNA for three months and are currently on placement. George feels that staff within the placement have not made them feel welcome, and at times have been at best unhelpful. George decided to ask the practice assessor for support as this was affecting the learning opportunities being made available. The practice assessor responded to George's concerns in a defensive way, suggesting that George has not tried to fit into the team and that this is the learner's responsibility, not that of the practice assessor or wider team, as team working is an important part of practice. George does not say anything after this but is ignored with a request for help with moving a patient where two people are identified as required.

George decides to approach the link tutor from the university to express concern that the team do not seem to 'like' them, and that this is affecting their ability to work together in the best interests of the patient. The tutor comes back and raises a concern within the university as when they discussed the situation with the education lead within the placement; they suggested George was trying to work without the team, thinking they were better than the team.

In the case study, you can see how an experience can be viewed depending on the perspective of the individual – there is a disconnect between George and the team for whatever reason. George has tried to address this as they see it; however, the response gives a different point of view.

Activity 5.9   Reflection and critical thinking

Reflect on the case study and answer the questions:

What impact do you think this had on George?

What impact do you think this had on the team?

What impact would this have on the patient experience?

What are the implications in this scenario and how you think it could be resolved?

Would you act on this as Duty of Candour, freedom to speak up or whistle-blowing?

An outline answer is provided at the end of the chapter, but remember that each situation is different, so your experience in clinical practice may differ.

Following the Francis Report (Mid Staffordshire NHS Foundation Trust Public Inquiry 2013), Lord Willis was asked to complete a review of healthcare and nurse education and training (Health Education England, 2015). In this report, they identified a gap between the training, knowledge and skills of HCAs and registered nurses, as well as recognising that the role of the registered nurse had evolved. This resulted in nurses undertaking more challenging roles as the complexity of patients' co-morbidities increased over time. In the past, Enrolled Nurses had filled some of the gap; however, that training and registration ceased in the 1990s. The outcome of the Shape of Caring Review was for a role to be introduced to bridge the gap between the nurse and HCA, to provide education to a level that supports the role of the registered nurse.

As discussed earlier in the chapter, the standards for the nursing associate were developed by the NMC, to be read alongside the standards for registered nurses, to ensure both are clear on role boundaries. These standards were aimed at future proofing the nursing profession, so that nurses were equipped with the knowledge and skills that would be demanded of them as their role continues to evolve, and complement the standards for the nursing associate. It is therefore important that when you read the nursing associate standards you also read the registered nurse standards, so you have a clear understanding of the different expectations of each role. As the nursing associate role has become embedded within different care environments, many have seen the opportunity for development of the role to enable and support different areas within practice. There have been discussions on the role within primary care, with different challenges identified for GP practices in comparison to other healthcare environments on the scope of practice for the role (Topping, 2023). One area of practice that has actively identified learning and competencies is critical care (Critical Care Networks, 2024), through a specific competency framework for nursing associates in adult critical care. This allows the nursing associate to achieve additional competencies to ensure that they are able to practise safely in this environment.

The key for you as a registered nursing associate is to ensure you remain within the scope of your practice as agreed locally, working within the limitation of your knowledge and skills, ensuring those you work with are aware of your ongoing developmental needs.

Chapter summary

In this chapter, you have identified the differences between responsibility and accountability, looked at the role of the NMC (2018a) *The Code, Standards of Proficiency for Nursing Associates* (NMC, 2024a), *Standards of Proficiency for Registered Nurses* (NMC, 2024b) and *Standards of Student Supervision and Assessment* (NMC, 2024c) to explore the roles and responsibilities involved in supporting learners in practice. The way these work in conjunction with each other should help you see where your role and responsibilities sit within your area of practice. The fact that the nursing associate role is evolving and requires competency development, supported through appropriate policy and education, has been emphasised. The background following the Francis Report and the Shape of Caring Review demonstrate how important speaking up is within practice, with the 6 Cs supporting positive approaches to care. The role of the Duty of Candour, freedom to speak up and whistle-blowing policies has been discussed to support you raising concerns, whether for your colleagues or your patients.

Activities: Brief outline answers

Activity 5.3 Critical thinking (page 70)

What responsibility does Julie have in this situation?

Julie has responsibility to inform the nurse that they lack knowledge and competence in using equipment to move patients.

What responsibility does the nurse have?

The nurse must ensure that Julie does not attempt to use the equipment and ensure training is provided and competence checked before expecting them to use it.

Who is accountable if Julie uses the equipment incorrectly?

If Julie informs the nurse they are not competent to use the equipment but the nurse requires them to go ahead and use it, the nurse is accountable.

If Julie does not inform the nurse, then Julie is accountable for their actions.

Activity 5.4 Critical thinking (page 72)

Read the standards of proficiency for registered nurses and nursing associates alongside each other.

How do you think these differ?

Platform 1: Being an accountable professional Nursing Associate Standard.

Nursing associates and registered nurses act in the best interests of people, putting them first and providing nursing care that is person-centred, safe and compassionate. They act professionally at all times and use their knowledge and experience to make evidence-based decisions and solve problems. They recognise and work within the limits of their competence and are responsible for their actions.

Registered nurses are also required to communicate effectively, act as role models, and are accountable for their actions. They must continually reflect on their practice and keep abreast of new and emerging developments in nursing, health and care.

Platform 2: Promoting health and preventing ill health.

Nursing associates play a role in supporting people to improve and maintain their mental, physical, behavioural health and well-being. They are actively involved in the prevention of and protection against disease and ill health, and engage in public health, community development, and in the reduction of health inequalities.

Registered nurses' role includes a broader requirement around health and well-being of people, families, communities and populations that includes global health.

Platform 3: Nursing associates provide and monitor care, where registered nurses assess needs and plan care.

Registered nurses prioritise the needs of people when assessing and reviewing their mental, physical, cognitive, behavioural, social and spiritual needs. They use information obtained during assessments to identify the priorities and requirements for person-centred and evidence-based nursing interventions and support. They work in partnership with people to develop person-centred care plans that take into account their circumstances, characteristics and preferences.

Nursing associates provide compassionate, safe and effective care and support to people in a range of care settings. They monitor the condition and health needs of people within their care on a continual basis in partnership with people, families, and carers. They contribute to ongoing assessment and can recognise when it is necessary to refer to others for reassessment.

Platform 4: Nursing associates focus on working collaboratively in interdisciplinary teams to communicate effectively within this.

Registered nurses focus on providing and evaluating care through taking the lead in providing evidence-based, compassionate and safe nursing interventions. They ensure that the care they provide and delegate is person-centred and of a consistently high standard. They support people of all ages in a range of care settings. They work in partnership with people, families and carers to evaluate whether care is effective and the goals of care have been met in line with their wishes, preferences and desired outcomes.

Platform 5: Improving safety and quality of care through monitoring people's experiences, identifying risks to safety. They put the best interest of people first, ensuring they meet preferences and personal needs.

Registered nurses lead and manage care teams, provide leadership by acting as a role model for best practice in the delivery of nursing care. They are responsible for managing nursing care and are accountable for the appropriate delegation and supervision of care provided by others in the team including lay carers. They play an active and equal role in the interdisciplinary team, collaborating and communicating effectively with a range of colleagues.

Platform 6: Nursing associates contribute to integrated care, including those with complex needs. They understand the roles of a range of professionals and carers from other organisations and settings who may be participating in the care of a person and their family, and their responsibilities in relation to communication and collaboration.

Registered nurses must focus on improving safety and quality of care, continuously monitoring the quality and improvement of care through assessment of risks to safety or experience and take appropriate action to manage those, putting the best interests, needs and preferences of people first.

Platform 7: There is no platform 7 for nursing associates. Registered nurses coordinate care, through leadership in coordinating and managing the complex nursing and integrated care needs of people at any stage of their lives, across a range of organisations and settings. They contribute to processes of organisational change through an awareness of local and national policies.

In your area of practice, what actions or activities do you think could be considered that of the registered nurse and that of the registered nursing associate?

The registered nurse will plan and coordinate each day at work, delegating to others within the team, including nursing associates. They will be primarily responsible for managing all care needs of patients or service users are met, addressing any risks as they occur, responding to changes or concerns where these are raised. The registered nursing associate will receive delegated tasks and manage their workload, reporting back to the nurse in charge. They work with a range of other professionals within the setting, including delegation of tasks appropriately, reporting any changes or concerns to the nurse.

Activity 5.6 Work-based learning (page 74)

Think about your own experiences of learning so far. What has been the most helpful learning experience and which has been the least helpful?

Most helpful – where the nurse asked what I already knew and then demonstrated and explained what they were doing at the same time. Afterwards, they reflected with me so I could see that I understood and was able to link to theory as well.

Least helpful – the nurse assumed that I had a foundation knowledge of working in a hospital ward but all my work and previous experiences have been in the community.

I was really unsure of myself in the clinical environment, but they were impatient with me, telling me I had to get on with it, even though I had never done any of these things before.

What made these helpful or unhelpful?

Helpful – the nurse asked and worked with me. Unhelpful – assumptions on my experience, knowledge and skills and impatience with me so that I felt undermined and lacked confidence for much longer than I might have done.

What would have made a difference to make your learning a more positive experience?

If they asked me what I knew, what I felt I needed to learn and worked with me.

What actions can you take to address this?

I could tell them but I am not sure if I could. I could talk to another nurse or my tutor/mentor/practice assessor.

How can you use this experience when you are required to supervise and support a learner in your practice area?

I will make sure that I work with someone to understand what they already know and what they feel they need to learn. I would encourage them to participate in new experiences alongside me until they, and I, felt they were competent enough to complete activities independently. I would use questions and verbal reflections to understand where they are in their learning within the environment.

Activity 5.7 Reflection (page 75)

Reflect on the learning opportunities you have experienced so far to identify both positive and negative experience.

Identify the barriers to your learning experience and whether anything could be done to overcome these.

Think about what you could do differently to gain different experiences.

Learning in home placement has been positive; I know the team and they know me and they are really supportive and want me to learn. I feel this has helped me to feel more confident as they believe in me. This contrasts with my first placement experience. I was very anxious as in a completely different care environment and I was worried I wouldn't manage. The practice assessor and supervisor were both busy on my first shift, so I was placed with an HCA. This helped me get a sense of the environment, the routines and different approaches needed, for example with recording physiological observations. This helped me get a sense of the area so when I was able to meet with my supervisor later in the day, I was able to let them know how different the area was and I was pleased to have spent time with the HCA. They were surprised that I saw this as a positive experience and we worked together to identify the areas of practice that were completely new to me, so they could ensure I was supported in learning these first. So, although my initial feelings were that I was not welcome or important, in fact, it helped me identify what I needed from the placement.

Now consider when you have or need to supervise others; this may be a new member of the team or another learner.

Having this experience has helped me to think about new people within my own practice area; the importance of making them feel welcomed. I can explain that we want them to learn about the environment and the daily routines so they have a good sense and can then be integrated within the team more effectively. By making time, even if only a few minutes, I can communicate and check in to be able to adjust what they are doing to support their learning.

This is linked to the importance of role modelling; if you have a positive approach to your learner, they are more likely have a positive approach when they have a learner.

Activity 5.9 Reflection and critical thinking (page 79)

Reflect on the case study and answer the questions:

What impact do you think this had on George? George has expressed they feel unsupported and unwelcome; they may interpret this as being because they are a SNA, or they may feel they are being discriminated against due to their nationality.

What impact do you think this had on the team? The team may feel defensive as they perceived George to be apart from the rest of the team, unresponsive to requests for support with tasks or directions for completion of delegated tasks.

What impact would this have on the patient experience? The potential is for patients to either not receive the care needed in a timely way as the team seek support from someone else, or left if George does not respond to their needs as they are unable to do so alone.

Consider what are the implications are in this scenario and how you think it could be resolved. There may be implications around George's practice; however, there could also be concerns around discrimination due to difference.

Would you act on this as Duty of Candour, freedom to speak up or whistle-blowing? This would depend on the specific scenario; however, where care has been omitted, this should be reported as a near miss under Duty of Candour, with the patient being given an explanation, an apology and information on what happened as a result.

If George is being discriminated against, this could also be raised as freedom to speak up as they feel this is the cause of the issue.

Annotated reading

4NHS England (2022a) Freedom to speak up online training is available through e-lfh, which requires an account to be set up through your employer. This link takes you to the information page: https://portal.e-lfh.org.uk/Component/Details/666118

NHS England (2022b) Our NHS People Promise was developed by those at the heart of working in the NHS to respond to the needs of all who work in the NHS, to be valued as an employee to enable consistent quality of person focused care to be delivered. This link takes you to the webpage: www.england.nhs.uk/our-nhs-people/online-version/lfaop/our-nhs-people-promise/

NMC (2019b) Guidance on using social media responsibly will enable you to ensure you operate within the requirements. These should be used alongside your employer and education provider guidance. Available at: www.nmc.org.uk/standards/guidance/social-media-guidance/read-social-media-guidance-online/

NMC (2019c) Professional Duty of Candour link to slide set outlines the NMC perspectives of the Duty of Candour as it applied to nurses, midwives and nursing associates./www.nmc.org.uk/standards/guidance/the-professional-duty-of-candour/

NMC Caring with confidence videos are a useful resource to support putting into practice the key points they identify as being fundamental to quality nursing care. https://nmc.org.uk/standards/code/code-in-action/

Chapter 6

Transitions and professional identity

NMC (2024A) *STANDARDS OF PROFICIENCY FOR NURSING ASSOCIATES*

Platform 1: Being an accountable professional

1.8   Understand and explain the meaning of resilience and emotional intelligence, and their influence on an individual's ability to provide care.

1.15   Take responsibility for continuous self-reflection, seeking and responding to support and feedback to develop professional knowledge and skills.

1.16   Act as an ambassador for their profession and promote public confidence in health and care services.

Platform 4: Working in teams

4.1   Demonstrate an awareness of the roles, responsibilities and scope of practice of different members of the nursing and interdisciplinary team, and their own role within it.

4.2   Demonstrate an ability to support and motivate other members of the care team and interact confidently with them.

Platform 5: Improving safety and quality of care

5.9   Recognise uncertainty and demonstrate an awareness of strategies to develop resilience in themselves. Know how to seek support to help deal with uncertain situations.

Chapter aims

- Identify the challenges faced when transitioning into a new role.
- Consider transitions at different stages of professional development.
- Understand the processes involved in change through change theory.
- Explore the impact change has on professional resilience and identity.

Introduction

This chapter will explore what you can expect from the process of change – from starting the nursing associate programme, through transition between year 1 and year 2 of your studies and transitioning into qualified practice. When you start something new, it involves change, which creates uncertainty – uncertainty about what will be expected of you, what you will be doing and whether you will be able to do it. To apply for the nursing associate programme, you must have had a belief that this is something you can achieve, but the reality when you actually start studying and working in a new way can feel overwhelming. Those who have supported you, whether family, colleagues, managers or friends, will create expectations, whether real or perceived, which can create pressure. The unknown requirements of academic study at Foundation Degree level, particularly if you have had difficult learning experiences in the past or not experienced higher education learning before, can also create anxiety and stress which undermine your confidence. You will see how this process of change may impact on your resilience and professional identity and explore ways in which you can manage transitions to enable you to succeed at different stages of your learning that can support you throughout your career.

Transitions in life occur all the time; however, recognising they can be stressful and challenge both your resilience and self-confidence is an important step in understanding the process of change that you are going through. It can feel like you have no control, but understanding what occurs when you experience a change, the emotions and the impact these have, can help you put strategies in place to guide you through difficult times. Remember, transition is a temporary state and you will adjust how you approach and manage yourself over time – allowing yourself that time to adjust will be the first step. Transition begins with the anticipation of change, this may be a mixture of feelings; excitement, anxiety, looking forward or fear all at the same time to create an emotional roller coaster. This continues until you have some stability – you have made the adjustments and managed your emotions and feelings to feel secure in your new 'place' (Darvill et al., 2021). This process has a number of different stages – understanding the stages can help through recognition of the stage and anticipating how to enable and manage the next stage.

Case study: Vicky part 1

Vicky has been working in primary care for 6 years and enjoys the role but during the last personal development review, Vicky's manager suggested that applying for the nursing associate as an apprentice would be a good opportunity for progression into a more involved role. Following the application and interview, Vicky has been accepted onto the programme at the local university. Despite feeling confident within the practice environment, feelings of doubt start to cause anxiety with the realisation that this is an academic programme and will involve writing essays. Vicky struggled at school, with teasing by peers because of slow reading in class. During careers information events, teachers suggested healthcare or hair-dressing as a non-academic option and after looking at both, Vicky decided that healthcare looked more interesting as there were different options and areas to work in. Before the interview, Vicky had not really thought about what would be involved as being an apprentice suggested this was learning while working; however, the university has sent information to Vicky on some reading that could help to prepare for the start of learning. This has triggered feelings of anxiety.

Understanding theory: Rites of passage

Rites of passage was first identified by van Gennep (1960) who explored the role of transition within society and for the individual. These transitions involve movement from one age to another, one occupation to another or from one group to another, recognising that although each experience is unique to you, there are patterns or similarities across different societies and cultures in experiencing transition. Through recognising these patterns, the rites of passage were identified and broken down into three distinct and separate stages: Rites of separation; Rites of transition and Rites of incorporation.

Separation

Separation involves you being removed from the safety of your existing situation, your 'comfort zone', as you are ending your current way of living or working. At this point, you may experience feelings of apprehension, enthusiasm and an eagerness formed from what you know or understand about the new situation you are moving into. You may look forward to your new situation as an SNA, second year SNA or registered nursing associate.

Transition

Transition is highlighted as occurring in the early months of your new situation, but is also considered the most challenging period of transition. During this time, you may start to doubt your choices about the new situation as you are unfamiliar with the ways things work or the expectations required, feeling out of your comfort zone. The uncertainty of this can lead to feeling that you are not ready for this new situation and possibly cause you to think you are alone in this. Over time, the expectations and demands being made of you will result in you starting to recognise what you need to do to help you adapt to this new situation.

Incorporation

Incorporation is when you settle into your new situation, recognise your new identity, or you are accepted by a new group, and it is a gradual process that may take some time. During this stage, you will start to feel more comfortable and confident with expectations, requirements of your role, responsibilities or routines based on your new knowledge or skills. You are moving into a new comfort zone.

Case study: Vicky part 2

Vicky's manager picked up that Vicky was not feeling quite right and in a conversation asked what was causing the anxiety. Vicky did not disclose the challenges experienced at school but identified worry about studying. To support Vicky, the manager arranged to meet Freida, an SNA from another practice that was coming towards the end of their first year of the programme. When they met, Frieda was able to let Vicky know about the different types of learning but also about the support that is available. They were reassuring but did not try and

(Continued)

(Continued)

hide the fact that there were expectations about reading and academic writing and how different that was. This is the separation stage.

Vicky started the programme a couple of weeks later and felt completely lost and like they were never going to understand what they were being taught. As part of their initial work, they had to look at their strengths and weaknesses to identify an action plan on how they would manage their needs. Vicky had a meeting with their allocated tutor and during the meeting became tearful. The tutor was patient and kind and made Vicky feel comfortable, so the experiences of school came tumbling out before Vicky had time to really think about it. The tutor was able to reassure Vicky, arranged for an assessment to see whether there were any undiagnosed learning needs, such as dyslexia, that could be supported by the university. They arranged regular tutorials to offer guidance and support and, over time, Vicky started to see that they were able to understand, they just needed things explaining to them in a different way. Once they recognised this, they were able to start to look at the learning needed differently and needed less support. This is the transition stage.

As Vicky approached the first assessment, although still feeling anxious, they felt they had done their best, they thought they understood and hoped they had done a good enough job on their assessment. When the results came out, Vicky had passed; it wasn't a high grade, but Vicky felt the achievement was beyond expectations, which buoyed their confidence for the next term. The following term, Vicky was able to join in the classes more, contributing to discussions with peers and became more involved in group work. Others in the class chatted about how they were feeling about the first assessment and the results they received and Vicky realised that although the feelings they experienced were unique to them, everyone had felt the same way. This helped a confidence that had not been experienced before and to feel accepted within the group, recognising they were sharing this experience and that they could support each other through this journey. This is the incorporation stage.

The process of transition van Gennep (1960) identified bases itself on three stages; since this was developed, others have explored the process to refine and break this down into smaller, more distinct processes, recognising that not everyone experiences transition in the same way, at the same stage, or manages to overcome and move into a new situation.

Understanding theory: The process of transition (Fisher, 2012)

Fisher (2012 cited in C2D 2021) looked at transition processes within a business context, but this can be applied to any profession and has been extensively used in healthcare learning. Fisher initially recognised that theory of change was usually thought about at an organisational level rather than looking at the individual experience, so he reversed this to think about the individual experience as a way of supporting people through the process of change. This transition process looks at the experiences involved as a journey (see Figure 6.1) with a range of emotions and responses you may, or may not experience along the way, which is why it is named the *personal transition curve*.

Progressing through the personal transition curve will be a unique experience to you. Others may have similar feelings or experiences; however, your previous experiences and how you respond will be unique to you and how you process and move through this will be unique to you. Being able to understand your own ways of being, your past experiences and how you perceive situations is partly how you will learn to navigate and manage change and manage those feelings of being outside your comfort zone. Any change, even a small one, can impact you in unexpected ways. This may involve conflict as your current beliefs and values are challenged and you contemplate new ones. To help you move through this process you need to know yourself; your perceptions of your past, the present and the future.

Activity 6.1   Reflection

Identify a previous change in your life that you have experienced.

Reflect on what you were losing as part of the change, and what you anticipated you would gain.

Think about how this affected you, what feelings you experienced and how you coped.

Now identify a change in your life that you are anticipating.

Reflect on what you are losing as part of the change, and what you anticipate you will gain.

Think about how this may affect you and what feelings you are experiencing.

Try to think about how you have coped with past changes to see whether there are any strategies you can use to help you through this experience of change.

This activity is a personal reflection, so there is no outline answer at the end of the chapter.

As you see in Figure 6.1, there are a number of emotions that you could experience during a transition. Exploring what these look like can help you recognise when you may be experiencing a particular stage of transition.

Anxiety

This results from recognising that you are unable to control, or understand. You are unable to see what the future will look like because the information you need to interpret what is required of you from this new situation is outside your knowledge or experience.

Happiness

Once you realise that others have similar perspectives to you, you can feel relief at not being alone in the experience, and that the change is going to happen. Whether you have had positive or negative experiences of change in the past, you hope, and possibly feel enthusiasm for the change as you expect a better future and see yourself succeeding. One challenge in this phase is that you may expect more from the change than is realistic and others may need to help you adjust your expectations, although you may not accept this perspective and reject this. This links to the NMC (2024a) *Standards of Proficiency for Nursing Associates* 1.5, 1.8, 1.15, 4.2 and 5.9.

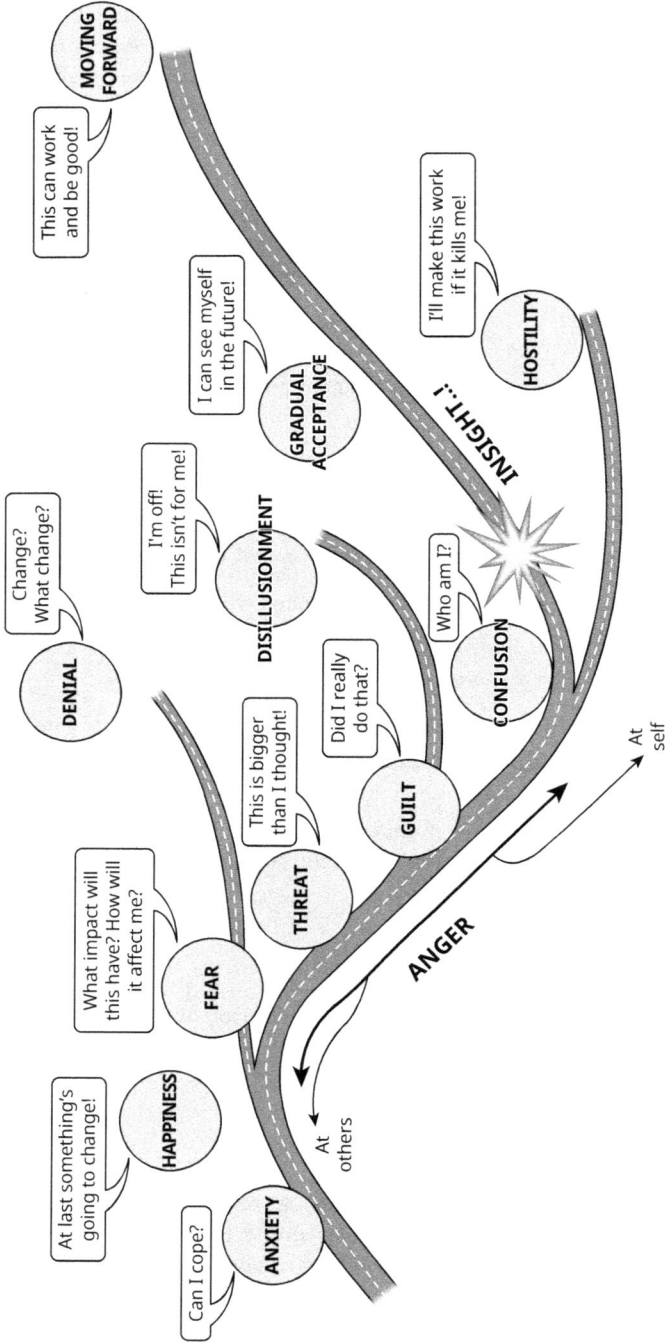

Figure 6.1   Fisher's personal transition curve

Fear

When you become aware of an imminent change needed to your beliefs, values or behaviour, you will need to behave in a different way, which can cause fear, with change to how you and others perceive you. You may believe that fundamentally that not much will change, you will still be you, but you are choosing this new situation and the new values, beliefs and behaviours that are associated with it. This links to the NMC (2024a) *Standards of Proficiency for Nursing Associates* 5.9.

Threat

You may become aware of fundamental changes to your core beliefs, values and behaviour and expect a major life change that has potential to change your future by creating different opportunities and how others will see you. You may feel uncertain that you will be able to respond or behave in the required way in this new situation as the responsibilities or rules are so different and you have yet to learn and understand the new ones.

Guilt

As you detach from your core perceptions of who you are and what is important to you, reflecting on your past and how you responded to change and start to consider the alternatives, you will start to create a new consciousness of who you are becoming. Examining your core beliefs, recognition of any inappropriate past behaviour can cause you to feel guilty when you acknowledge how these affected others.

Confusion (previously depression)

You may feel a level of uncertainty about what the future is going to be like, and how you are going to become a part of this new situation, that your motivation to make the change can be challenged. You may feel confused about what is needed, your thoughts and ideas compromise your sense of who you are, taking away your sense of identity but with no replacement. This can make you feel unsure how to behave, or what values and beliefs you need.

Gradual acceptance

When you start figuring out what the new situation requires of you, you can start making the changes to your behaviour, values or beliefs that enable you to consider the new situation and how you can fit into this. You will be trying out new ways of working to see what works to help you make the most of the new situation. This links to the NMC (2024a) *Standards of Proficiency for Nursing Associates* 1.5, 1.10, 1.15 and 5.9.

Moving forward

As the new situation is no longer so new you have found the best ways of working and are feeling secure and confident with the situation. You have found how you work best and are able to reflect on how you have changed. This links to the NMC (2024a) *Standards of Proficiency for Nursing Associates* 1.5, 1.8, 1.10, 1.15, 1.16, 4.1, 4.2, 5.9 and 5.10.

There are points where you may deviate from the personal transition curve, which may result in different short- or long-term success, although these are not so positive.

Disillusionment (Deviation 1)

You may feel that the beliefs, values and behaviours that are important to you conflict with the new ones required. The changes that you need to make feel contrary to what you feel is best for you. It may be that you recognise that this is not for you, the demands being made are too great. This can demotivate you and create dissatisfaction with the situation, resulting in you withdrawing mentally or emotionally, possibly just doing the bare minimum required. You may criticise the new situation, or physically withdraw from it. This conflicts with the NMC (2018a) *The Code* and NMC (2024a) *Standards of Proficiency for Nursing Associates*.

Hostility (Deviation 2)

You may have continued to try but ended up staying in your old ways of working and these are not being successful for you to adapt to the new situation, potentially ignoring or sabotaging them. This conflicts with the NMC (2018a) *The Code* and NMC (2024a) *Standards of Proficiency for Nursing Associates*.

Denial (Deviation 3)

You have not accepted that something needs to change, or that this will affect you, so you continue to behave as if the change has not happened, working in the same way you did before and ignoring information or evidence that contradicts your beliefs, values or behaviour. This conflicts with the NMC (2018a) *The Code* and NMC (2024a) *Standards of Proficiency for Nursing Associates*.

Anger

Sometimes, but not always, you may feel angry when you are moving through the personal transition curve. This is more likely in the early stages when you realise what you need to do to make the changes needed. Whether you feel angry, or the focus of your anger, will be linked to how much control you feel you have over the process of change and this may change as you progress through the process. You may feel that you did not have a choice and feel angry towards those you feel made you make the change, blaming them for the stress you experience as a result. Over time, the focus of your anger may change as the implications to you are recognised. At this time, you may turn your anger towards yourself for not controlling the situation better, which can in turn can make you feel guilty or confused and push you into the Guilt or Confused stage of the curve. This conflicts with the NMC (2018a) *The Code* and NMC (2024a) *Standards of Proficiency for Nursing Associates*.

Complacency

It was suggested that an additional stage was necessary, which Fisher has incorporated into the personal transition curve, either as a final or initial stage (C2D, 2021). As a final stage, you have survived the change, incorporated them into the way you work and got used to the new situation. You feel that you are confident with how you need to work, and anticipate that any new event is something you can manage and adapt to easily. You feel you know what the right decisions are and feel able to see what the future will be like. This may result in you being complacent, being relaxed about your approach to what you do, taking your foot off the pedal and not really paying attention to what is going on around you as you get on with things in the way you perceive them to be needed. You may have found the process of personal transition stressful and challenging but when you reach this stage you have forgotten all of that and cannot understand what others are making a fuss about.

Activity 6.2 Reflection and critical thinking

Reflect on the final suggested stage of complacency.

Consider which parts of the NMC (2018a) code of professional behaviours this potentially compromises.

An outline answer is provided at the end of the chapter.

Sometimes, you may not recognise which part of the personal transition curve you may be experiencing; therefore, being supported in the process of change is an important consideration. Although you may want to achieve this on your own, perhaps to prove something to yourself or others, having someone who can help you navigate this process effectively may minimise the challenges for you. This person needs to be able to share information or educate you on what you can do to enable you to achieve. This sounds easy but is often missed as your emotional responses take over and you fail to recognise the signs of anxiety, fear, happiness or threat for example, as discussed in Chapter 3 on resilience. This results in you reacting through complaining about the situation, or trying to keep things as they were as these are what you know and understand, rather than managing your emotions. This results in an increase in your experience of stress.

You may work through some stages quite quickly, where others may take more time; you may not even realise that you are in a stage unless you are reflecting regularly on the process. However, the theory proposes that this is a linear process, with each stage contributing towards the next, accumulating over time to create the depth of emotion experienced.

Case study: Vicky, part 3

Vicky's initial anxiety about returning to study and having to read and write essays had impacted on her sense of self as part of Fisher's first stage. This was the result of recognising what they were going to have to do, which is the fear or threat stage. This understanding led Vicky to feel guilty, and to an extent, depressed, as their self-belief system had been weakened.

One challenge that can occur is when you experience multiple transitions simultaneously. The cumulative effects contribute to you seeing this as evidence that supports any previous negative self-belief, perceived or otherwise. In the case study, Vicky had previous poor experiences at school that led them to believe they were not capable of writing essays or completing the reading needed for these – these would compound the anxiety and feelings of fear or threat they experienced. They may not have even realised they were within the happiness stage, as this may have been a fleeting emotion of elation they had been accepted onto the course, or relief they had started as they felt they had some input into their future and that things could turn out for the best. It is at this point that interventions to help you through the process of change can have the biggest impact as they have the potential to 'flatten' the curve through those that can help you through the process giving you the information you need, or you accessing the support you need. Essentially, you recognise that you do not need to do this on your own.

The personal transition curve has not undergone any experimental research on whether you will experience each stage in turn as outlined; however, the process is based on Kübler-Ross's five stages of grief (Kübler-Ross and Kessler, 2005). Research has shown that this process is not linear and that different stages can overlap; therefore, you may not experience all stages or experience them in the order in which they appear on the curve. Your **locus of control**, which is the level of belief you have on how much control you have over events in your life, whether these are caused by things outside your control, or whether you are able to control these yourself, will also influence your experience of transition (see annotated reading). Other influences will depend on how you perceive yourself, your previous experiences and how these contribute towards how you think about future transitions; however, it is important to recognise that much of this will occur in your subconscious. Reflecting on your experiences, particularly when you feel anxious, will help you recognise when you are in the process as well as where you are, with the way you respond dependent on how proactive you are at seeking and accessing support. The role of your personal resilience will also influence how you react and respond to the transition process, reviewing the activities from Chapter 3 and applying your transition experiences to these may help you identify strategies that can enable you to feel confident in overcoming some of the challenges you face through the process of change. As part of your ongoing professional development, reflection and a proactive approach to this will become embedded within your professional identity.

It is possible that you could feel disempowered, which may result in sliding down into the depression stage, compounded by feelings of helplessness. You may insist in working in the same way you have in the past, or follow through behaviours that in the past have resulted in failure or do not enable you to see things from a different point of view. You may want to deny that there is anything that needs to change, these all have a negative impact on you and your experience of change and this would require additional input to help others help you through the process; looking at what your past perceptions are, and how you see the future, what impact change has had on you in the past and how you coped with that, and helping you see what you may be losing and gaining as part of the change. These pitfalls can compromise your professionalism and how others view you as your professional identity needs to align with the NMC (2018a) *The Code*. Reflection at different stages of the transition process will support recognition and create opportunities; however, you may not always feel like you belong.

Imposter syndrome

Sometimes, you may want to make a change so decide to 'go for it' but when you start something new, you feel like a fraud, that you should not be there, or you do not deserve to be there. This is known as imposter syndrome, where you may decide that the reason you are there is pure luck or because others helped you, rather than something you have done to get you there, and that any setbacks are the direct result of your flaws or inadequacy within the context of the situation. This comes from a lack of recognising your own knowledge or competence as being the cause or reason for your success. Research into imposter syndrome in nursing shows that this can occur during transitions, feeling unprepared, as a result from stress, not having enough social interaction with others, come from a lack of self-compassion, uncertainty about your role or as a result of limited clinical experience (Edwards-Maddox, 2023).

Imposter syndrome is more common than you think; if you talk to others about their role or experience of learning, you are likely to find others who feel this way as well. Recognising you are not alone, sharing your experiences, giving and receiving positive feedback can all help develop and overcome imposter syndrome, although you may always carry some of those feelings within you.

Case study: Matt

Matt is a second year SNA who was home schooled and therefore did not achieve any formal qualifications. They had cared for a disabled parent throughout their life, focusing on this until early adulthood. During the COVID-19 pandemic, they had realised there was a whole world they knew nothing about and felt they wanted to experience. They spent some time researching what they could do, realising they had no qualifications and little life experience, they completed their functional skills in English and Maths online. Once the pandemic was over, they decided to move to a local town and managed to get a job caring for young people with disabilities, which they really enjoyed and gained satisfaction from. The manager of the care company suggested they could complete an apprenticeship as a nursing associate as a first step towards becoming a nurse.

Matt applied for and was accepted for the course and managed the first year quite successfully. During the final review meeting of the first year, they revealed that they felt like an imposter in the university, that they did not deserve to be there as they did not have the education that everyone else had and that they did not feel part of the peer group as a result. They were isolated and lonely as they had nothing in common with any of their colleagues or peers. This surprised the university staff and their manager, who had seen Matt as an able student and SNA; they were competent within the practical role, and had achieved well academically. However, Matt claimed this was just lucky and that the emotional turmoil created was making them feel burnt out and unable to continue. The tutor referred Matt to support services, who over time helped Matt unpack their feelings and the cause of these both in the academic and care environment. Matt was able to see that they had possibly more knowledge and experience of caring, having lived with this role for many years. During a class session, Matt talked to a few peers about their feelings and was surprised that their peers also felt the same way. They found it hard to believe Matt had no formal schooling as they viewed contributions made as being evidence of their own inadequacy. This developed into a support circle within the group, where they were able to support each other and then start to recognise their own contributions as being worthy through the positive feedback they received.

Another way of looking at imposter syndrome is to reframe this as your inner critic; you are likely to be your biggest critic. Thinking about constructive criticism rather than criticising can be completed through reflection to enable you to explore what you do, why you do something a particular way, whether there are alternative ways that may be better and what outcomes may result from changing your approach. Reflection and support are both powerful tools you can use to recognise and identify how to move forward, which in turn will help you manage your emotional responses and enable you to navigate transitions at different stages of your career. This is where using some of the learning from Chapter 2 can be utilised to support your ongoing development. The importance of recognising and managing your own needs cannot be stressed enough – the requirements of the NMC (2024a) *Standards of Proficiency for Nursing Associates* clearly incorporate concepts of resilience discussed in Chapter 3, vulnerability, reflection discussed in Chapter 2, and self-management as outlined at the start of the chapter. This is because they are associated with experiences of patient care – where you are less able to recognise and manage these for yourself, potentially this results in poorer quality of care for patients resulting from burnout.

Burnout is when you feel emotionally exhausted, you may be cynical about what you are doing, why you are doing it or what you are learning, which results in limiting what you can achieve. Your responses are less effective because you are experiencing chronic stress that is not being managed. This is an individual response that happens over a period of time; it can develop at different rates and can result in both physical and psychological symptoms (Maslach and Leiter, 2016). You may not recognise it until the symptoms start to take hold or you are open to reflecting on what the cause may be, although the cynic in you may not recognise this and blame others. Whenever you feel others are responsible, whether they are or this is your perception, you should take time to reflect on the situation and consider what impact your behaviour has on the quality of the relationships you need to maintain within the practice environment with both colleagues and patients. Regardless of who is at fault, as someone working towards an NMC registration, or holding a registration, you have a duty to address this. This will require an open mind to the cause and what needs to change; you are part of this process, even if it is others who were the initial cause. This may be difficult to address and you will need to consider accessing support through your employer or union to complete this process.

Hopes and fears

Everyone will experience hopes and fears, identifying these can support your preparation for transition at different stages of your life, both professionally and personally.

Activity 6.3   Reflection

Consider your hopes and fears for the different points of your learning journey.

What were/are your hopes and fears before you started learning?

How did/do you feel about transitioning from year one to year two?

What are you/might you be feeling when transitioning to become a qualified nursing associate?

You may be a qualified nursing associate about to transition to a new role or onto another programme of study, again, you will have hopes and fears involved with this that you need to identify.

Now think about what might support you with this, for example your clinical education team, tutors and other learning support teams at your education provider, family, friends, peers or a preceptorship programme.

Identify how long you should allow yourself with the transition process.

How often you can get together with those who can support you?

Can you spend time with different people who will be able to help you with different parts of your learning, both clinical and academic.

What opportunities are there to develop your knowledge, skills and experiences that can help you navigate any challenges you face?

What support you need with this?

How can you gain feedback on your performance?

How to continue to develop this?

Take time to think about how you reduce your feelings of stress.

What activities do you enjoy that will help you maintain a balance outside of clinical practice and learning?

Who can you make contact with? For example, how can networking with peers and colleagues help you with both managing your learning needs and gaining feedback for you to reflect on and what transferable skills do you have that can enable you with this process?

This activity is a personal reflection, so there is no outline answer at the end of the chapter.

Student top tips

This is student feedback on moving to year 2 of an SNA course:
It's ok not to know – just make sure you ask.

Spend as much time talking to patients/listening to patient stories as you can.

Do not avoid what feels scary – now is the safe time.

Take time to reflect on your practice experiences.

Make sure you are supervised until you feel ready to do something alone.

Remember to take breaks when you are supernumerary.

Be aware – very experienced people do not always know best.

Be tactful if challenging something.

Get bank experience if you can.

Transferable skills

Transferable skills are those that can be applied to different situations, and you will have a number of these that you can use to support you through transitions.

Activity 6.4 Reflection

Identify what transferable skills you have and how these may be able to help you with the process of transitioning into a new role or situation.

This activity is a personal reflection, so there is no outline answer at the end of the chapter.

Transferable skills are wide ranging and will be individual to you, particularly for clinical experiences; however, there are some fundamental skills that you are likely to possess. Recognising some of these can enable you to create a confidence where perhaps you do not always feel this when you are exposed to new situations.

Communication is something you may feel is a strength as you communicate daily with those you work with, patients, colleagues, family or friends. Taking time to think about how you communicate successfully will support you in transferring this to a new situation.

Teamwork is a key area of practice in health and care, even if you work independently in the community, you are still part of a team, working together to identify best working practices, supporting each other when faced with problems or challenges.

Empathy is the ability to listen and understand someone else's point of view, being able to be present in the moment.

Time management may be a big part of your life, with managing family, work and study. Recognising how you organise yourself or your workload and knowing what information you need to do this effectively will support you in managing your time well across different situations to enable continued effective patient care is delivered.

As you progress through your learning and practice experiences, you will be able to take new experiences to add to your existing ones. This accumulation of knowledge and experience will support you in managing transitions at different points in your career. Table 6.1 summarises transferable skills you may have and will develop as you progress towards qualifying as a nursing associate.

Table 6.1   Examples of transferable skills

Transferable Skills	Examples of what transferable skills
Communication	Face to face and telephone conversations, negotiating, influencing and listening
Team work	Sharing information, pooling skills, supporting colleagues under pressure, treating colleagues with respect
Management and leadership	Setting targets, taking responsibility for other staff, motivating people, delegating, training others, making evidence-based decisions
Planning and organisation	Setting schedules, making arrangements, monitoring progress towards targets, working independently
Empathy	Active listening, asking for feedback, dealing with complaints, defusing situations, tact and diplomacy
Time management	Prioritising workloads, multitasking, working under pressure, meeting deadlines, delegation
Taking initiative	Coming up with solutions and ideas for problems, coping with the unexpected

Chapter summary

This chapter has explored how transitions can affect you at different points in your career. The process of transition has shown there are different emotions and feelings that can be experienced, with Fisher's personal transition curve focusing on understanding what you can expect and how you may be able to access support to minimise the impact this has on you. Accessing support and enabling you to manage your needs to avoid burnout, including your own locus of control and the role of reflection in identifying and managing your needs to ensure you meet

NMC's *The* Code (2018a) and *Standards of Proficiency for Nursing* Associates (2024a) has been discussed. The negative impact of imposter syndrome highlighted this is experienced by others in healthcare practice, with ways of overcoming and reframing how you think about yourself as a management strategy considered. Reflecting on transitions and how you can negotiate these, things you need to consider and how you can utilise existing knowledge and skills conclude the opportunity for you to manage this process to enable you to continue to give safe, effective patient care as you are able to demonstrate resilience and maintain professionalism as you develop your professional identity.

Activities: Brief outline answers

Activity 6.2: Reflection (page 95)

Reflect on the final suggested stage of complacency to consider which parts of the NMC (2018a) code of professional behaviours this potentially compromises.

*The NMC code may be compromised through lack of self-awareness of attitudes and behaviours that could impact on working within a team, or being open to new **evidence-based practice**. 1.3 requires avoiding making assumptions; assuming the way I work is the 'right' way. 2.1 working in partnership; if I am not recognising that there is a new way of working, I may work alone which compromises this. It would also contradict 8.1, where I need to respect the skills and expertise of colleagues and potentially conflict with 8.2 around managing effective communication with them. As a team, we should work together to evaluate the quality of the care delivered within the team for 8.4 through 9.1 providing honest and accurate constructive feedback – if I am complacent and believe my way is the way, it may not be constructive or accurate. I need to consider feedback given to me, with complacency, 9.2 would not be adhered to and 9.3 where differences of opinion occur would also be neglected. This links to 20.3, where I need to be aware of my behaviour and how this affects others behaviour and potentially create a poor role model linking 20.8 and compromise my own mental or emotional health with 20.9 which in turn neglects requirements of 20.1, upholding the values and standards within the code.*

Annotated reading

Watch this YouTube video by Dr Tracey Marks on Locus of Control to help you explore your own way thinking. This will help you recognise areas you may need to consider developing to move from an external locus of control towards a more internal locus of control: www.youtube.com/watch?v=0mKDhwk4a_g

This link includes a useful downloadable guide from the RCN for newly qualified nursing associates that will support your transition to registered practice: www.rcn.org.uk/membership/Existing-members/Nursing-support-worker-members/Newly-Registered-Nursing-Associates-guide

Chapter 7

Chapter 7

Employability skills

NMC (2024A) *STANDARDS OF PROFICIENCY FOR NURSING ASSOCIATES*

Platform 1: Being an accountable professional

1.7   Describe the principles of research and how research findings are used to inform evidence-based practice.

1.15 Take responsibility for continuous self-reflection, seeking and responding to support and feedback to develop professional knowledge and skills.

1.16 Act as an ambassador for their profession and promote public confidence in health and care services.

Platform 4: Working in teams

4.1   Demonstrate an awareness of the roles, responsibilities and scope of practice of different members of the nursing and interdisciplinary team, and their own role within it.

4.8   Contribute to team reflection activities, to promote improvements in practice and services.

4.9   Discuss the influence of policy and political drivers that impact health and care provision.

Platform 5: Improving safety and quality of care

5.2   Participate in data collection to support audit activity, and contribute to the implementation of quality improvement strategies.

5.10 Understand their own role and the roles of all other staff at different levels of experience and seniority in the event of a major incident.

Platform 6: Contributing to integrated care

6.1   Understand the roles of the different providers of health and care. Demonstrate the ability to work collaboratively and in partnership with professionals from different agencies in inter-disciplinary teams.

Chapter aims

- Explore differences between practical and theoretical knowledge and their relationship to professional practice.
- Consider Benner's novice to expert theory and your own place in this.
- Make links between knowledge and experience to deliver safe and effective care.
- Understand how application and interviews can be supported through recognising your strengths and weakness within your practice.
- Explore resources available to support application processes.

Introduction

Wherever you are in your career, starting out as an SNA, or working towards your first or subsequent registered roles, it is useful to reflect on your knowledge and experiences to try to link these to highlight your strengths, weaknesses, opportunities and barriers (SWOB). You may find it useful to review Chapter 1 activities, particularly on your SWOB analysis, to periodically review your career progress. Strengths are useful in demonstrating your capabilities, whereas weaknesses show self-awareness and the ability to recognise your limitations and suggest openness for further learning. Recognising how everyone can move from a knowledgeable practitioner to someone who lacks the relevant knowledge and experiences, can help support your confidence to change and take up opportunities within new areas of practice. With the nursing associate having a unique scope of practice across the four fields of practice – adult, mental health, child and learning disability, this provides ongoing opportunities to identify different knowledge and skills that can increase your employability through understanding how these transfer between different roles and areas of practice.

When you set out on a new career path, it can feel exciting but also quite daunting, particularly if you are unsure about what you want to do in the longer term. As part of your learning, you will be exposed to new experiences that may influence future choices; using these to explore different opportunities requires confidence in your knowledge and skills, something you may not always have. In this chapter, you will explore how you can use reflection explored in Chapter 2, your existing and developing knowledge and experiences to enable you to explore your transferable employability skills to plan a career strategy. Exploring different areas of practice, the knowledge and skills that are required, can help you make informed decisions about your career both as you are learning and beyond registration. To support this, you will be thinking about the process involved in job applications and interviews so that you can adequately prepare and give yourself the best chance of success. A career in health and care offers many new and exciting opportunities, with these evolving over time to reflect the changing health and care landscape. By preparing at this stage in your career, you create a confidence in matching your experiences, maintaining and furthering your knowledge to enable you to follow a sometimes very different career path to your initial plans. This may include progression towards becoming a registered nurse.

The unique role of the nursing associate

The role of the nursing associate is a unique one, in that it allows you to work across a range of different areas without having to complete specific education for that discipline. This is a significant contrast to being a registered nurse, as nurses are only able to work within the individual discipline, adult, child, mental health or learning disability, in which they are registered. This uniqueness offers you opportunities to move between disciplines and areas of practice, although to be able to do this you will need to be able to demonstrate the knowledge and skills you have that you are able to transfer to the new discipline. There are many skills that are transferable, the key here is that you are able to articulate your skills and how you are able to use these within the new discipline. This requires you to have a high level of self-awareness, honesty about your experiences and knowledge, as well as confidence to explore possibilities. Revisiting your strengths, weaknesses opportunities and barriers discussed in Chapter 1 can help you think through different elements of experience and knowledge, to recognise how these can apply elsewhere. You may also want to revisit Chapter 6 on transitions. This relates to NMC (2024a) *Standards of Proficiency for Nursing Associates* 1.1; 1.15; 4.1; and 5.10.

There are different types of knowledge: the knowledge you gain from direct experiences in practice, the knowledge you gain from learning through your education provider and the knowledge of how to put what you have learnt in theory into practice. You will be used to this through ongoing assessments that use case studies and your reflections within practice assessment documents, where you have demonstrated links between theory, such as new knowledge of anatomy and physiology.

Experiential knowledge

Experiential learning stems from transformation of knowledge through experience as a process where knowledge is the outcome of understanding what is needed. In Chapter 2, you explored Kolb's (1984) experiential learning cycle, the process involved in learning through experience and how you assimilate this within practice. It may be useful for you to revisit this to remind yourself of the process. Now, at this stage of your learning, you need to be able to think about what you have learnt within practice and how this relates to other areas of practice to help you identify your transferable skills.

Activity 7.1   Reflection and critical thinking

Identify the knowledge you have acquired through your practice experiences, what can you do now that you could not do before and how has this changed the way you work, for example through the way you communicate with patients or your colleagues.

Why do you think your approaches have changed, what do you know that you did not know before?

What can you take from this to use in another area of practice, such as paediatrics, learning disability practice, mental health or social care?

This activity is a personal reflection, so the outline answer at the end of the chapter provides guidance only.

Learning through experience is just one element of your learning journey, by understanding what you have learnt in practice through experience will help you to link knowledge gained through academic learning to consolidate your knowledge as being based in theory and evidence, essential elements for nursing associate practice – you will need to be able to articulate what you are doing and why you are doing it in a particular way.

Academic knowledge

When you start academic learning, you will be focused on what you need to learn to achieve the requirements of the course, although one of the challenges can be recognising the purpose of what you are learning and how this links to what you do in practice. You may feel that you know how you do something and that your knowledge is intuitive, stemming from experience as discussed in the previous section. This is called tacit knowledge, you just know what to do but you may not be able to explain why you need to do it (Johannessen, 2022). When you are in an academic learning situation, you will be gaining the underpinning knowledge from theory and the evidence base that will help inform why you do what you do the way you do it. Sometimes, theory can be challenging to understand but hopefully you have grasped the concepts, some of which have been discussed in previous chapters. Now all you need to do is join the dots to show you know how theory and evidence guides your practical approaches. This is where reflective practice can be of significant benefit, as you are able to think about what you are doing and why you are doing it in a particular way, and as part of your analysis and evaluation, you can use evidence and theory to explain these.

Activity 7.2   Reflection

Identify some theories or new academic knowledge you have gained and match them to some practical skills you have developed. You may want to format this as a table, with your skills or experiences in one column and the academic knowledge sources that relate to them in another as outlined at the end of the chapter.

This activity is personal to you. An outline answer is provided at the end of the chapter, but remember that you are unique so your own experience is likely to differ.

There are some more obvious examples you could think about, such as how anatomy and physiology help you understand basic physiological observations in a patient – how a slower or faster heart rate is manifesting in your patient, why they have a slower or faster heart rate and what action prescribed medication can have on the heart rate, are examples of knowledge that can be applied to practice. Other theory may involve communication theory, how emotions are communicated between a patient and yourself as a practitioner using Mehrabian's (1972) communication theory to help you understand that perhaps what the patient is saying does not match what you are interpreting from their communication with you. It can be helpful if you list new knowledge and then link these to the practical aspects of your role, see Table 7.2 within the activity answers at the end of the chapter.

Connecting experiential and academic knowledge

Using the exercise in Activity 7.2 can enable you to start making the links between your experiential knowledge, tacit knowledge and academic knowledge to help you embed this within your practice. In doing this, you are then able to consider the skills and knowledge you have, to identify how this could be transferred to another practice environment. The process involved is rooted in reflective practice and it will be worth revisiting Chapter 2 if you still find reflection challenging to complete.

When considering alternative areas of practice, taking time to explore the job description, the essential and desirable skills, using this process to link what your current knowledge is to the job description, will demonstrate to you what you do know. Hopefully, this will allow you to feel confidence in your knowledge and skills. Where you are unable to match up the knowledge and skills, this creates an opportunity to fill the gap through further learning, another strong skill valued by employers – being proactive in recognising both your strengths and weaknesses, addressing your weaknesses, can be a strong 'selling' point for you during interviews. This demonstrates your attitudes and behaviours towards learning, meeting the requirements for a particular post or area of practice, as well as demonstrating fundamental aspects within the NMC (2018a) *The Code* 6.1, 6.2, 13.5, 19.2, 20.1, 20.6, 20.8, 22.2, 22.3, and 1.1, 1.7, 1.15, 1.16, 4.1, from the *Standards of Proficiency for Nursing Associates* (NMC, 2024a).

You may feel that where you have a lot of experience and then applied your new knowledge, your practice is at the top of your ability. This may be a point where you start to consider alternatives; however, this can also create uncertainty, as discussed in Chapter 6.

Understanding theory: Benner (1982) novice to expert

When you become knowledgeable and skilled within a particular area of practice, others can start to rely on you, you feel confident in your practice and do not necessarily feel you have any more to learn in that particular environment. Benner (1982) recognised this within nursing practice and developed a scale for practitioners to measure where they are within their current practice, see Table 7.1. This scale may have featured in your practice assessment document or may have been used as part of your practice assessments. Benner recognised that nursing involved tacit knowledge as discussed earlier; however, as nursing roles became more involved and patient needs more complex, the need to be able to articulate why, giving a rationale and thinking through options for managing situations became imperative for safe clinical decision making. At that time, nurses learnt from one another through observation, trying and practising until mastered. The obvious disadvantage of this approach is if you are taught a procedure incorrectly, you then work in the same way without really understanding that it is incorrect and possibly unsafe. Learning within practice may still have a strong element of observation, trying and practice, and you may feel more confident learning through this kinaesthetic learning by doing process. However, nowadays, this is the point in your practice where you need to be able to articulate why you are doing something in a particular way and whether there is an alternative, more effective way. This is called critical thinking, a term you will recognise from feedback on your academic assessments.

(Continued)

(Continued)

Table 7.1   Benner's model

Novice	This is when you are a beginner with no practical experience of how to apply new knowledge and skills in unique situations.
Advanced Beginner	This starts as you begin to use your previous experiences intuitively.
Competent	This is when you have developed the ability to prioritise and utilise aspects of situations that are most relevant. You are able to think consciously and analytically as you explore why rather than just do. You start to feel that you are achieving skills and you are efficient and organised in planning your work.
Proficient	You are able to look at situations holistically, spending less time and energy thinking through and planning. You now know what needs to be done without someone telling or asking you to do it.
Expert	This is when your experience and intuition are highly developed as you are able to bring together theory and practice without conscious thought. And able to explain this to others.

A key feature of Benner's model is that this depends on the situation rather than being an attribute that you possess. You are situated in a place where you have a definable amount of knowledge and experience.

Activity 7.3   Critical reflection

Using Table 7.1, identify where you are in the novice to expert process for your normal area of practice.

Now reflect on your first day as an SNA, where were you at that time and has this changed?

Now think about each placement you have completed, where on the novice to expert spectrum were you at the start and end of the experience?

This activity is a personal reflection, so there is no outline answer at the end of the chapter.

Novice to expert in practice

When you consider moving into a new area of practice, you will be in a new situation and therefore will need to recognise that you will move from being a more confident and competent practitioner to one who is starting to learn new things again. It does not matter how long you have been qualified, or how much experience you have; when you move to a new situation, you will become either a novice or advanced beginner again. As a novice, you have yet to be able to apply new knowledge and skills in this unique new experience. You are likely to need general rules to understand what is expected of you; you may not be able to be flexible to meet the needs of the environment and your ability may be limited. As you develop an understanding of the new situation, you start to process the rules and guidance, using the experiences you have gained to start to recognise the context of the situation and respond more intuitively, although you will be using these alongside principles and checklists to ensure you apply those learnt rules. As you develop a stronger grasp on the rules and context you can then start to develop competence. Here you can start to use your analytical skills to prioritise your work and filter out what is more or less important at a particular time. Your thought processes will be conscious, you still need to think about what you are doing, how and why, as you start to master the knowledge and skills needed. This is when you are becoming efficient in your work and feel a sense of responsibility, reflecting on what went well but also what can be improved in your practice.

As you progress through the competence stage to being proficient, you can see situations holistically, picking up cues as situations change and are able to respond to these changes appropriately, without having to spend a lot of time thinking about what is needed, why, what other options are, as you understand what is needed within the situation; you are able to be flexible in your approaches. Being an expert in nursing can be more difficult to pinpoint; you will have lots of knowledge and experience, you will have strong intuition based on being able to identify the specific theoretical knowledge and apply this within your practice without really having to think about it, but would be able to explain your decision making to others. At this stage, you would be finding solutions to clinical issues, thinking innovatively; thinking outside the box to find ways forward based on theory and evidence.

Self-assessment of where you are within Benner's framework can be challenging; this is where reflective practice and feedback from others continues to support and enable you to recognise where you are. The role of honesty in your self-evaluation is important, but so is balancing this with not allowing your inner critic to be unduly harsh and undermine your self-confidence. As an SNA moving towards or into registered practice, it is important to be aware of the levels of responsibility required to make effective clinical judgements to ensure you remain within the scope of your practice. You may underestimate the preparation required for your new role and need support to manage the challenges faced when you first qualify and register with the NMC, and therefore you may feel you step back within Benner's novice to expert framework. This is because you are moving from a learner, who is competent, or even proficient within the scope of learner practice, to being accountable for your practice and your clinical decision-making as a registrant. Clinical decision-making in practice requires a good awareness of how you manage yourself. If you have an approach to everyday life, you are likely to also have a similar approach within your clinical practice.

Activity 7.4 Decision-making

From this list, identify how you approach and achieve goals, challenges and tasks in everyday life.

I view challenging problems as tasks to be mastered.

I develop deeper interest in the activities in which I participate.

I form a stronger sense of commitment to my interests and activities.

I recover quickly from setbacks and disappointments.

I avoid challenging tasks.

I believe that difficult tasks and situations are beyond my capabilities.

(Continued)

(Continued)

> *I focus on personal failings and negative outcomes.*
>
> *I quickly lose confidence in my personal abilities.*
>
> *For each phrase you identify with, consider what actions you could take to try and develop yourself and consider how these may impact your clinical decision-making.*
>
> *An outline answer is provided at the end of the chapter, but remember that each situation is different, so your experience in clinical practice may differ.*

Ways of managing the change from SNA to registered practice includes asking your practice assessor, practice supervisor, your manager or a trusted colleague to provide you with positive feedback on your successful completion of tasks and if they can help you reflect on your knowledge from theory and the evidence base. You could also use the template in Chapter 1 to complete a SWOB analysis to apply academic knowledge to practice. These will help you to increase your confidence and recognise where you have gaps that you need to address. When you develop an awareness of your approaches to managing situations, and how you can change your way of thinking to embrace change, you can apply these principles to new opportunities that you may wish to consider. When you have this, you can start to consider what, and how, you present yourself within a personal statement for job applications.

Job applications

Preparing yourself for job applications is a starting point. If you have a clear idea of your areas of interest and how your knowledge and skills may transfer to that area, you can start looking at adverts to explore how you can match what is wanted to what you are able to offer. Most adverts will contain a brief outline of the organisation, area and expectations of the role, although these may be generic, or lack specific points for you to make links with. The Job Description and Person Specification will have more concrete details about the knowledge and skills needed, but researching the area will also give you ideas on what you can link within your application to match your knowledge, experience and skills. These will also highlight areas that may be developed into questions you may be asked at interview. Additionally, organising an informal interview or visit to the area will also help you prepare. Remember, this is about whether the job is right for you as much as whether you are right for the job. High-lighting key skills, experience or personal attributes the job description requires can be used to see what you have and whether these match; think about some specific examples from your recent practice that can help you demonstrate the experience rather than relying on general examples. These may be separated into essential or desirable skills, knowledge or attributes – if you do not meet all the essential criteria, you could identify this in your SWOB to create an action plan on how to address this. It is also worth talking to the contact linked in the advert to find out whether it is worth still completing the application. You can always ask for feedback, which is advisable, as this allows you to address any issues within your application.

Personal statement

Once the main application form is completed, you will need to write a personal statement. This is your opportunity to demonstrate how you match the skills, knowledge and experience identified in the job description and person specification. Never assume because you work in a particular area that the person reading your application will know what you do, the knowledge you need or the skills you may have – make it explicit in your personal statement. This may include current and previous roles both in and outside health and care services or life experience such as caring for a relative or any projects you have completed – remember your previous experiences can create knowledge and skills in different ways that can be transferred across. Think about the academic and practice learning you have completed to become a nursing associate and how that relates to the role you are applying for. Identify whether you are involved in any professional networks such as the RCN forums – see annotated reading. Have you been included in any research or audit development, advocacy or perhaps you have an activist/champion role within your organisation, for example equality and diversity champion, infection control link worker, or well-being champion among other things. If you have not been actively involved and these opportunities are available, it is worth thinking about applying as they add extra value to you as an employee as well as demonstrate your commitment to further your knowledge, skills and experiences. When you have an area that you have no experience to relate to, think about how you would manage that situation and use an example of what you would do in a particular situation – it is better to be honest about what you have not got and demonstrate how you could address this, again this shows self-awareness, honesty and integrity as well as a willingness to learn new skills which support application of the NMC (2018a) *The Code*.

Structure of your personal statement should use the order in the person specification, making it clear which points you are discussing; use the same words and language. Take care as there are often many requirements outlined but you do not want your statement to be too long or too short. This is so the person reading them for shortlisting people for interview can clearly see how you meet the requirements set out. It will also minimise the risk of missing an important point out. Remember, your written communication will also be assessed; make sure your spelling, punctuation, grammar and use of professional language are to a good standard; follow all instructions and organise your application logically – this shows your ability to present yourself, your examples or evidence in a succinct way that retains the essence of who you are. If you can get shortlisted for interview, you have done well as this shows you have been able to match your knowledge, experiences and skills to the requirements for the role.

Case study and critical thinking: Juliet

Juliet is writing a personal statement for a job as a children's and young people's community nursing associate. They have not worked within paediatrics before but enjoyed a few days in community paediatric clinic during their final placement. They decide to use this experience alongside the specific learning from the course to demonstrate the essential and desirable requirements within the job description and person specification. The extracts below demonstrate two approaches to this.

Example 1

I have recently qualified as a nursing associate and registered with the NMC. During the course, we covered the life span to ensure knowledge of the underpinning theories that are necessary for working with children and young people, people with learning disabilities and mental health needs at different times of their lives. I applied child development theory in an assessment through a case study that linked attachment theory to the behaviours being observed in an adult I had cared for. I experienced a placement in a community paediatric clinic where I worked with children and young people. My written and verbal communication skills have developed through written academic assignments, with further feedback from my practice assessor on improvement of my written documentation and verbal handovers.

(Continued)

Example 2

During my final placement within the community paediatric clinic, I developed a passion for working with children and young people with a range of health needs. I was able to work with children who had communication difficulties, as I learnt some basic Makaton sign language. My practice supervisor delegated redressing a surgical wound on a 6-year-old child with Autistic Spectrum Disorder. The parent, also present, commented that this was the first time the child had allowed someone who they did not know to work with them. During this process, I explained to the child and the parent what I was doing, sometimes using Makaton pictures where I did not know the specific signs, asking my practice supervisor for advice as needed. I felt that the wound was not healing well, through reflection together, I referred to a Dr for review. I then followed up with the community nursing team to visit the child at home. This mirrors my experience of working within a surgical unit, where discharge of patients to the community often requires referral onto community nurses or social care. This process is an area that I recently supported through audit of referrals, where gaps in information were highlighted. I worked as part of the project team to create a flow chart of essential information required. Colleagues fed back through my practice assessment document on my communication and involvement with this as I spent some time researching evidence for development of the protocol.

1. Which of the examples is stronger?
2. Why do you think that is?

An outline answer is provided at the end of the chapter, but remember that each situation is different, so your experience in clinical practice may differ.

Activity 7.4   Research

Locate a job description and personal specification for a nursing associate role that you may be interested in. Using this and the STAR principles, develop a personal statement.

S – Situation (when and where did this happen?)

T – Task (what did you have to do?)

A – Action (how did you do it?)

R – Result (what was the outcome?)

This is a personal activity; therefore, no outline answer is provided at the end of the chapter.

The STAR model is an RCN (2025) resource for members; therefore, the annotated reading can only be accessed if you are a member. There are other union websites and resources – Unison, Unite and Community are other UK unions that will have resources available (see annotated reading). It is advisable to join a union as this can offer resources, advice and support for pay awards, support when something goes wrong, as well as offering learning packages to support your ongoing CPD requirements, as discussed in Chapter 8.

Developing interview skills

When you have successfully secured an interview, your next focus should be preparing for this and thinking about how you can sell yourself. This is something that nurses are not known for doing, as skills are difficult to define and articulate. Once you identify your skills, you need to be able to articulate these to sell yourself, especially why you are trying to move into a different area of practice. Use specific examples to support you, as these provide evidence. It is also where your research on the area and organisation can shine through. Remember, you can learn specific clinical skills but what sort of nursing associate, or what values and behaviours you possess, need to come across clearly so the interview panel can evaluate them.

One way of approaching this is to create some possible questions based on the job description and person specification. You can then practise possible questions, prepare your answers, practise talking through them out loud, or ask someone to ask you questions so you can practise your interview technique.

Body language

Your body language will communicate a lot of information to the interview panel and how you manage this can be influenced positively or negatively by how confident you feel about being interviewed, the role, your own knowledge and skills (Ganguly, 2017). You may lack confidence, which can impact on your body language but also your ability to think and communicate verbally in the moment. Your own body language communicates with you as well as others; when you feel powerless, you make yourself smaller and when you feel powerful, you make yourself bigger. The hormones testosterone and cortisol are linked to this process, with greater levels shown to be present in people who perceive themselves to be powerful. This has led to understanding that your body can influence your mind, and this then changes your behaviour, which then changes the outcomes you experience.

If you lack confidence in interviews, there is a useful technique to help you manage your anxiety – see annotated reading YouTube video Fake it Till You Make it (Cuddy, 2012). This focuses on preparing yourself physically and mentally before you attend an interview – using a private space, make yourself bigger by expanding your arms up and over your head, taking deep breaths for around five minutes. This increases the release of the hormones that make you feel more powerful, which in turn can increase your confidence at interview, or other situations such as presentations. Whether you are successful or not at an interview, it is useful to ask for feedback so that you can learn and develop. Ask specifically about your answers, but also about how confident you came across and whether there is anything you can continue to work on with your interview technique.

Chapter summary

This chapter has looked at experiential and academic knowledge, and how this is needed to work together for safe, effective clinical decision-making. Through re-evaluation of your knowledge and skills, you have explored how you can match these to enable you to develop a career strategy or plan. When looking at a specific role that you may wish to consider, using your strengths can help you make links between your knowledge and experience and what a job wants from the candidate. How you use your weaknesses to address gaps in knowledge and experience can support continued learning and professional development as a proactive

(Continued)

(Continued)

thinking approach. There were links to Benner's novice to expert framework. The use of transferable employability skills can then be used to identify specific examples from your experiences to complete a personal statement as part of a job application. How to prepare for interview, developing confidence and gaining feedback on your interview technique can be used to build a stronger performance in future.

Activities: Brief outline answers

Activity 7.1 Reflection and critical thinking (page 105)

Identify knowledge you have acquired through your practice experiences, what can you do now that you could not do before and how have you changed the way you practice, for example through the way you communicate with patients or your colleagues. *Since starting the SNA programme, I have improved my documentation as I am able to understand more of the terminology used and the structure of what I write has improved. When I communicate within the MDT, I am able to explain my thoughts clearly and this has been acknowledged by colleagues through feedback in my practice assessment document.*

Being shown new clinical skills, such as drug rounds, has helped me think about things like why the nurse should not be disturbed during the drug round that I had never really understood when I was a HCA. Being able to take blood through venepuncture is a practical skill that I have learnt and through practice feel confident in completing as I have had several patients where it was difficult to obtain the sample.

When I talk to patients, I am able to think about what their needs are as I am able to get to their level, making sure I am listening and checking that I have understood what they need, whereas before, I would assume I knew what they needed but this wasn't always right and some patients may not have had what they needed from me.

Why do you think your approaches have changed, what do you know that you did not know before? *My approaches have changed because I have been working with my practice supervisors and watched how they work. They have also questioned me why they are doing something or why I am doing something in a certain way. This has helped me to think through the decisions that I am making. What I now know is that there are sometimes lots of options, many may be positive but some may not be positive for a particular situation or a particular patient and therefore, I need to make sure I am aware and working with the patient rather than making assumptions.*

With venepuncture, just having the exposure to different people has helped me develop confidence in taking blood; I explain what I am doing and why so they are aware of everything, gaining continued consent when it is difficult to obtain a sample.

What can you take from this to use in another area of practice, such as paediatrics, learning disability practice, mental health or social care?

Even if I have not worked with a child, someone with a mental health need or a learning disability, the principle of not making an assumption still holds true; I need to be able to communicate clearly with the person and if needed, get help in understanding what they are communicating with me. I can think through the different options or ask those with more experience to check whether I have correctly understood and come to a conclusion that fits with that person's needs as this is a fundamental skill.

Venepuncture on a child or someone with a learning disability may need more time and attention to their understanding of what is happening so they are able to be still while I get the sample. The understanding of how different people respond, their anxieties and fears are all real for them, so being able to be efficient is important to minimise distress, which is where lots of different experience really helps.

Activity 7.2 Reflection (page 106)

Table 7.2 Example of a completed reflection on skills, experiences and new academic knowledge sources gained. *Remember, these are unique to your own experiences, so are likely to differ.*

Table 7.2

Skill or experience	Academic knowledge source
Educating patients	Public health theory; health coaching theory; health literacy
Medication management	SafeMedicate©; anatomy and physiology
Documentation	Academic written work; health care laws and guidance
Verbal handovers	Presentations

Activity 7.4 Research (page 109)

From this list, identify how you approach and achieve goals, challenges and tasks in everyday life.

I view challenging problems as tasks to be mastered.

I develop deeper interest in the activities in which I participate.

I form a stronger sense of commitment to my interests and activities. *Because I feel a commitment to my interests, when I am interested in my studies I put more effort into them. This gives me better grades and positive feedback that increases my confidence in my knowledge. I can then feel confident when I am in practice that I know and understand a relevant theory or aware of the evidence – or how to find the evidence to make sure I am working within best practice. To continue my development, I could expand the areas of practice I am involved in, which will continue to strengthen my practice.*

I recover quickly from setbacks and disappointments.

I avoid challenging tasks. *When I am faced with completing a new skill, I feel daunted so I avoid it when I can. This is slowing down my practice and frustrating my practice assessor, who has identified that I need to be more proactive with practising practical clinical procedures. It also means that I am not becoming more skilled in completing skills that I need, which also affects my confidence on shift at times. I need to tell my supervisor how I feel – I could ask them to make me practise with them until I feel confident when I am learning a new skill.*

I believe that difficult tasks and situations are beyond my capabilities.

I focus on personal failings and negative outcomes.

I quickly lose confidence in my personal abilities.

For each phrase you identify with, consider what actions you could take to try and develop yourself and consider how these may impact your clinical decision-making.

Annotated reading

These resources can offer advice and support to prepare for job or course applications and interviews:

NHS Jobs is a central source of information for all staff across the NHS. It outlines roles and opportunities, as well as provide information and advice for job applications. www.jobs.nhs.uk/candidate/search/advice/making-successful-applications

RCN trade union www.rcn.org.uk/*The RCN has a range of resources that support with job applications, continued learning and a number of professional forums that you can get involved in. These can promote your professional profile in job applications.*

Unison trade union *offers advice and support for job applications and includes a range of resources for ongoing professional development.* www.unison.org.uk/at-work/health-care/representing-you/

Unite trade union *offers advice and support for job applications and includes a range of resources for ongoing professional development.* www.unitetheunion.org/what-we-do/unite-in-your-sector/health-sector

Community trade union *offers advice and support for job applications and includes a range of resources for ongoing professional development.* https://community-tu.org/

Watch this *YouTube video by Amy Cuddy, Fake it Till You Make it. It explores the research and science behind power and success, with some excellent tips on how you can use your body language to increase your confidence.* youtube.com/watch?v=RVmM eMcGcoY

Continuing professional development and NMC revalidation

NMC (2024A) *STANDARDS OF PROFICIENCY FOR NURSING ASSOCIATES*

Platform 1: Being an accountable professional

1.1 Understand and act in accordance with The Code: Professional standards of practice and behaviour for nurses, midwives and nursing associates, and fulfil all registration requirements.

1.15 Take responsibility for continuous self-reflection, seeking and responding to support and feedback to develop professional knowledge and skills.

1.16 Act as an ambassador for their profession and promote public confidence in health and care services.

Platform 4: Working in teams

4.7 Support, supervise and act as a role model to nursing associate students, healthcare support workers and those new to care roles; review the quality of the care they provide, promoting reflection and providing constructive feedback.

Chapter aims

- Identify how continuing professional development (CPD) supports career progression.
- Explore the role of locus of control and how this can influence your ongoing development.
- Consider the role and purpose of revalidation with the NMC.
- Understand the role and responsibilities of a registrant confirmer.
- Create a 5-year personal development plan.

Introduction

As you progress towards the end of your learning, you will need to start thinking about what progression looks like for you. This could be continuation in your role as a nursing associate in an area that is familiar, or you may decide to branch out and explore other areas of practice or progress to a registered nurse. Whatever your decision around this may be, it will entail continuing professional development (CPD). Not only will CPD enable you to progress, it allows you to maintain your registration with the NMC through revalidation. Combining your work from Chapter 7 on strengths and weakness identification on other roles and areas of practice, with opportunities for CPD and meeting NMC revalidation requirements, will be explored to enable you to review these requirements as part of your ongoing career planning, exploring where you want to be in 5 years' time. This does not mean you have to follow this path, but will help you identify a focus for CPD opportunities to plan and work towards your longer-term goal.

Why is CPD important?

CPD is something the NMC requires all registrants to complete; understanding why this is important can help you focus on the choices you may have available to you once you are qualified and registered with the NMC. This is so you can remain up to date with current knowledge and best practice; knowledge and evidence can change as new research and evidence emerge. This enables you to remain safe and effective in the care that you deliver to patients and service users throughout your career as this can span a number of decades.

There will be several aspects of your life that will influence your career choices, some of which you have control of, others, you may not be able to control. This chapter considers some actions and activities that can support your decision-making, hopefully to expand your vision of what is possible through lifelong learning.

You may consider your career in different ways, through matching your knowledge and skills, areas of interest, preferences or interests you have with areas of practice that require or attract similar people. You may have heard the term 'psychometric testing'; this is based on the premise that the person is 'suited' to a particular type of role or team through analysing your personality, aptitudes and critical thinking skills. However, it does not give the whole picture, only an insight into possible responses to a situation.

Sometimes, you may think that careers are influenced through external factors, viewing opportunities as more open or closed to others, for example ability, social class or educational background. Other times, you may think of careers as a cyclical process, where you explore ideas, gain confidence, identify a role or practice environment you may be interested in, maintaining a role until circumstances or personal motivations change. You can be left feeling 'here we go again' a new start, the honeymoon period, then disillusionment resulting in making another new start – remember the personal transition curve discussed in Chapter 6 that explored the different stages of change. To avoid falling into this, consider the role of planning your career, thinking through what you want and how you can achieve it. Not only does this motivate you, it will enable you to develop a strategy and work towards defined goals using SMART goals (Doran, 1981) identified in Chapter 1.

Case study: Mamoud: Part 1

Mamoud has worked within adult learning disability community services as a nursing associate for four years. They have enjoyed their time, but feel they have achieved all they can within the environment and consider themselves 'expert' within the Benner (1992) novice to expert framework. They enjoyed their placements within a local acute trust and decide to start exploring roles that become available. Despite their thoughts on a change in direction, they are unsure what will be the best direction for them at this time, having recently become a parent for the first time. As the main income bringer for the family, they would like to progress further in their career. Initially, they find there are three nursing associate roles, one in paediatrics, one in a surgical assessment unit and one in a complex frailty unit. They would also like to continue their professional development to become a registered nurse one day, but unsure whether they want this within learning disability or adult.

Developing a career

There are many ways that you can think through what you want for your future, for example, you could think of your career as a story 'Once upon a time . . .'. Building a narrative about your career, where, when and how you want this to develop is one way of identifying the different stages you will need to work towards. Considering past experiences and how these support or direct the direction your career aspirations may take can also be useful as you will draw on the transferable skills discussed in Chapter 7.

Activity 8.1   Reflection

Consider the following point:

Is building a logical career 'narrative' important? If so, to who?

Where did your narrative start; how did you get into working in health and care?

What you are doing now, how will that influence your narrative now?

What are you thinking of doing next; does that extend your narrative in the same or a different direction?

. . ...and your plan for after that?

This activity is a personal reflection, so there is no outline answer at the end of the chapter.

The reality is that you may have some wonderful plans for your future. However, the opportunities, knowledge and skills needed to enable that to be successfully navigated can sometimes be elusive; there may not be a role available for you to progress into, your personal circumstances may change and you may not have the capacity to dedicate the time to studying as you hoped, any number of things can get in the way. It can sometimes be easy to take the path of least resistance and resign yourself to settling for what is available, to feel like you have no control over some factors that are needed for your plan to succeed.

Understanding theory: Locus of control

The concept of having a locus of control was developed by Rotter (1966) and relates to how you feel a sense of agency – the sense of control you feel you have to influence your thoughts and behaviour. There are two locus of control types: an internal locus of control where you feel you influence your own abilities, actions or mistakes; or an external locus of control, where you think that chance, environmental factors or others actions are impacting or influencing your life without you having control over these. You will not have just one or the other; this is a spectrum and you are likely to have some of each in varying degrees. There can be genetic factors, childhood experiences, learnt behaviours and attitudes from child-hood caregivers that influence which type of locus of control you have.

One caution on external locus of control and the research – the research is not extensive, with additional limitations on the research study participants. As in much research, participants are from Westernised, middle-class backgrounds. Cultural psychology, the approach to this research, shows that findings may not be applied to East Asian culture or those from a lower socio-economic background. These backgrounds are linked to less opportunities for choice, although this is a generalisation. Therefore, those from backgrounds who have experienced reduced opportunities for choice, integrity and self-control, rather than a personal influence or control over the environment, may be more relatable. This requires self-awareness and under-standing your own cultural upbringing to recognise if this applies to you but are equally important for meeting the NMC (2024a) *Standards of Proficiency for Nursing Associates*.

Further research has identified that when Western middle-class people are faced with reduced choices, they want the restricted item more. This contrasts with those from working-class backgrounds, where choices are already limited, as they tend to accept what is available. Sheehy-Skeffington and Rea (2017) go further to assert that the decision-making of those who grow up in poverty focuses on the here and now, as they are unable to see how the future could be, therefore they are likely to find forward planning and motivation to follow through on these plans much more challenging. Therefore, agency, which underpins research on perceived control, is not necessarily applicable in these cultural contexts, particularly where people's life circumstances provide fewer options, as this influences their long-term expectations.

Locus of control

Although there are some factors that you cannot control, as discussed in Chapter 6, you are able to identify specific challenges and consider how to address through changing your attitudes or behaviours, to ensure you practise safely and effectively to meet the NMC (2024a) *Standards of Proficiency for Nursing Associates* 1.1, 1.15, 1.16 and 4.7. Being able to understand your own locus of control will help you explore how you approach making any changes needed.

It is important not to confuse your locus of control with your desire to control; these are conceptually different things within your personality, although there will be a relationship between these. For example, you can control how often you look to see whether a role becomes available by checking the jobs bulletin each week, but you cannot control when a role will become available. Your internal locus of control would recognise that you are able to apply for a role that you are interested in as you have checked the bulletin regularly, rather than it just being luck that a role was advertised when you happened to look at the bulletin, which would link to a strong external locus of control. Basically, these differ in how much control you believe you have and how much control you want to have; you may want to have control but feel you have not got that level of control. Research has linked those with a stronger external locus of control – the lack of control, to having a low desire for control, and this suggests you are more likely to experience 'lows', believing you have more control than you really do. This approach has been linked to gambling and superstitious behaviours; you will know yourself whether you have a tendency to take risks, or hold superstitions. The mismatch of the amount of control you want, and the amount of control you have, could have a negative impact on your psychological well-being; therefore, developing yourself, your self-awareness and resilience, as discussed in Chapters 3, 5 and 6, will help you work towards changing your outlook.

Case study: Mamoud: Part 2

Mamoud discusses the options available with his family, as they feel it is important this decision is supported and does not place them all under undue pressure. Their partner recognises that Mamoud is stagnating and restless, stating that they will support them in whatever decision they make, including whether they decide to wait to have another child until Mamoud is a registered nurse, however long that takes. Mamoud feels they have control over their situation and matches their existing skills to each of the roles that are available. They also research options that may be available for completing the registered nurse qualification. They realise that this could take three or four years to achieve so they need to make some decisions, identifying what they have control over and what they do not.

Using a strengths and weakness analysis, Mamoud identifies areas of practice that align to each role. Through this, they see they are able to use transferable skills to all three settings, however, the strongest area is the surgical assessment unit. To assist with this, they contact the unit and ask if they are able to visit for an informal discussion and the potential they have in applying for the post. The unit manager agrees to meet Mamoud, although expresses concern over the time since Mamoud last completed some clinical skills. Afterwards, Mamoud feels they were lucky to be able to see the unit manager as they are able to set some SMART targets to address some of the challenges to secure an interview, such as knowledge of medications used and general conditions that may be referred to the unit. They also identify which clinical skills they have continued to use regularly in their current post, which would require additional competency assessment and whether opportunities exist within the current setting to complete these.

Activity 8.2   Case study analysis

Identify which are the areas of the case study that show an internal locus of control.

Identify which are the areas of the case study that show an external locus of control.

An outline answer is provided at the end of the chapter.

Internal model of control

Perceived control, like locus of control or self-efficacy, can be explained as a basic internal working model you develop to map opportunities for control. This map is built on implicit expectations resulting from your experiences, but it is not made up of guidelines, rules, regulations or probability. It uses emotions and motivational conviction about your *personal force*, your ability to create an *apparent reality* that includes opportunities to realise the outcomes you want to achieve, but also any threats, dangers, or challenges to these by avoiding unwanted outcomes. These internal assessments contribute to whether you are ready to take action, through guiding your choices, the effort and the approach you take, and sustaining your efforts.

How you perceive the control and influence over actions you take in life will result from the amount of control you feel you have, competence you have, and how you plan for outcomes that are either unwanted or unexpected, through contingency planning. Control would be represented by asking 'Can I influence this important outcome in the direction I desire?' Contingency and competence would reframe this question to 'Do I have what it takes to get what I want?'. If both contingency and competence are necessary conditions for achieving control, then if either are absent this would result in its loss. If you believe the outcome is unlikely, because outcomes are based on uncontrollable causes, like powerful others, luck, or chance, or are simply unknown, or incompetence based on perceived lack of will or ability or access to other causes, will undermine your control.

There is some evidence where a sense of control influences outcomes such as education, health and societal involvement. These are linked more positively with those who have an internal locus of control, suggesting you are more likely to be successful, healthier and happier than if you have an external locus of control. To explore your own locus of control, there are a number of websites that use free quizzes to assess this – see annotated reading.

Activity 8.3   Locus of control quiz

Complete the locus of control quiz identified in annotated reading. Following the test, reflect on the outcomes highlighted – do you agree or recognise these?

An outline answer is provided at the end of the chapter, but remember that you are unique, so your own experience is likely to differ.

You can use the outcomes identified in Activity 8.3 to understand your own personality and approaches to life, how you are influenced and what impact this has both on your practice and the opportunities available to ongoing professional development. You can also think through how you can change your attitudes or approaches in small ways to place yourself 'in charge' of your life where you can, through revisiting the activities in Chapter 6.

Developing a five-year plan

To help you with your career and making the most of opportunities available, it can be useful to develop a longer-term plan. As outlined in Chapter 7, analysing your strengths and weaknesses, any opportunities that are available and barriers to your development is an excellent starting point as this will allow you to consider what actions you can take. Remember to apply the SMART (Doran, 1981) approach discussed in Chapter 1, breaking these down into smaller, more achievable short-term goals that help you work towards your larger goal – *eat an elephant bite by bite* is a popular saying to help overcome feeling overwhelmed by the task you set yourself.

S Specific – what is the specific aim of your plan, for example, in 5 years' time I will be a registered nurse. In order to achieve that, you will need to break it down, for example, identify where you can access the opportunity, whether you can be supported by your employer, whether you meet the entry requirements, when the course starts each year and which year you plan to start.

M Measurable – There will be different points in time you can measure where you are with achieving your overall goal that are linked to the smaller actions outlined. Set yourself regular intervals to review and reset actions to keep you on track.

A Achievable – Consider what you need to do to achieve the longer-term goal; for example, you may continue to access professional journals to help you retain your academic reading skills, or you may participate in a project in practice that can be written up for publication that will support your academic writing.

R Realistic – are your goals realistic to achieve with the available resources; for example, if your employer has a limited number of places for the BSc pre-registration nursing apprenticeship they can support each year, what is the likelihood you will be able to be supported. There may be additional activities, such as participating in a champion role, or completing further training to promote your own case; these can then be added to your specific shorter-term goals.

T Time-bound – what do you want to achieve when, be specific, set reminders in your phone or in your calendar to review where you are in your plan. Try writing yourself a letter to open the following year that outlines your aspirations, what you have achieved in the last year and what you plan for the year ahead. This is a nice way to start a new year through remembering how you felt, what you thought and reflecting on how far you have come over that time. This can also help you think through what you need to do and plan your CPD activities.

Case study: Mamoud: Part 3

Mamoud writes a detailed five year plan that outlines ambitions to move to the surgical unit, and after 12 to 18 months, to be supported accessing the degree nurse apprenticeship. In this outline, they identify fear of not securing the post desired and outline the SMART actions they need to follow to maximise their chances, but also another option they have considered if they are unsuccessful. The plan includes extending their family as they progress towards registering as a nurse. Mamoud feels the plan is realistic, but fears arise from others not seeing the potential in them, something they feel they have no control over.

Mamoud applies for the role in the surgical assessment unit but is unsuccessful. The manager feedback suggests Mamoud continues to address the gaps in knowledge and skills by working some bank shifts at the hospital. Six months later, another role is advertised in the unit and Mamoud applies again, this time, they are successful. When they start at the unit, the manager shares the positive impression Mamoud created by the proactive actions taken to enable them to gain the knowledge and skills required; they encourage further learning within the Trust and suggest application for the BSc Degree Nursing Apprenticeship the following year. Mamoud and partner welcome their second child two weeks after qualifying as a registered nurse. The following year, Mamoud reads the letter written while working in Learning Disability services. They cannot believe so much has changed over the time; it took longer than they hoped but they made it happen within the five years. Mamoud considers what their ambitions might include for the next five years and decides to start the process again so they can plan their CPD and potential opportunities for further progression.

Continuing professional development (CPD)

CPD is described as the way that you continue, keep and enhance your knowledge and skills through continued learning and development. This is to ensure you deliver safe and effective patient care throughout your career, particularly through keeping up to date with the latest research, guidance and legislation. There are many ways you can achieve CPD without having to undertake formal courses, although if you wish to continue developing a career, this is a desirable option. CPD is made up of a number of different options ranging from conference attendance, formal accredited learning to social media interaction among other activities.

Structured learning, either through in-person or online resources is the most commonly considered CPD activity, with a range of options available through a number of sources, not just universities. Your employer will be able to advise whether there is an opportunity for CPD funding; this is usually dependent on the course, the course costs and duration. You may be able to get released to attend or complete learning, or you may be required to complete this in your own time. It can be helpful for you to consider carefully what you will gain from an accredited course, whether you can afford the time and/or cost involved, and what gains you will achieve from it. Even if this is for your personal interest, that is a gain, as you are fulfilling a desire of your own, and all learning will contribute to your long-term career.

Workshops are a good way to gain practical knowledge and skills, particularly if you are considering a change in direction as this can show your interest, as well as develop your skills. It is also a good place to meet and network with other practitioners; here you may be able to find out about other areas of practice, show an interest and possibly arrange a visit, all of which shows your proactive approach, as seen in the case study with Mamoud, that can set you apart from other applicants if you decide to go down that route.

Peer review activities are helpful as you can gain 360° feedback on your practice; think back to Chapter 1 and the Johari Window (Luft and Ingham, 1955) activity, to use this feedback to gain insight into how others perceive your practice and where or how you can enhance this. This activity is a good use of your time and free, you can complete with any number of people from different disciplines within your area, and is something you can repeat to demonstrate your growth in a particular area based on feedback – also excellent for reflection for NMC revalidation.

Reading and reviewing publications can enable you to demonstrate keeping yourself up to date with guidance for your area of practice; it will also help you retain the skills to read more complex articles, including research. This will help you if you decide to return to more formal learning later as these skills are quickly forgotten! Your department may subscribe to a particular journal, or you may have colleagues who have subscriptions they are prepared to share. If you work for the NHS, public health, social care, an Integrated Care Board or GP practice you should be able to get an OpenAthens account through NICE (2024) that gives you free access to a number of journals. If you work for a different organisation, your application will be assessed for eligibility. To access this, you will need to register with your NHS email account and give the name of your organisation – see annotated reading.

Enquiry-based research may sound daunting but if you are involved in clinical audits, or supporting colleagues in gathering data for service improvement or a research project, then you can utilise this. If the project is to be published, consider getting involved with writing up data; again, this will enable you to retain academic writing skills for future formal learning, as well as an opportunity to add to your portfolio.

Coaching as discussed in Chapter 4, and mentoring in a specific role, either as a participant or as the coach, strengthens your knowledge and skills in sharing new knowledge and adds value to you as a member of a team. This can also be strengthened through using the Johari Window to gain feedback on your coaching skills or approach to learning in practice to provide another strong subject for reflection for NMC revalidation.

Conferences are a sought after opportunity; they are often expensive but there are some that are free or offer early bird prices. They can either be in person or virtual; the catch for in-person conferences can be location of the conference, with the addition of travel and accommodation costs, although the benefits in terms of networking and gaining learning and insight from other practitioners is worth considering. Employers may agree to fund some or all of the costs but a good way of securing this is to try and participate in the conference. Submitting a proposal for a poster presentation on an activity you have been involved in, either audit, service improvement or a research initiative with others can be a valuable learning experience and can be completed as either an individual or multiple authors, which would help you with the first experience of this process. Each conference has its own requirements, often focused on a theme, so this does require preplanning, looking for a conference that fits with the theme of your work project. There are specific conferences for nursing associate practice that could be a good starting point for you to explore. There are numerous benefits of conferences, through networking with colleagues, learning from outstanding practice, understanding how practice changes and develops, exploring opportunities, how local policies and governance can support practice, reflect on national developments, learn from lived experience of practitioners, as well as the support for CPD for revalidation evidence.

Social media is now recognised by the NMC as a source of learning, although you need to ensure your engagement with this is in line with their, and your employer's, social media guidance. X, formerly Twitter, and other social network platforms have professional accounts that you can engage with that are managed by professionals who want to network more extensively. Participating in a social media 'chat', which is a conversation that takes place using short messages, can enable you to explore professional issues that are important to you and can count towards your participatory learning hours. It is also a useful way to follow organisations, such as the NMC, RCN, Health Foundation, Kings Fund to name a few, that enable you to keep up to date with current topics, resources and publications as they become available. If you decide to do this, it is worth creating a separate professional account where you can create a biography about your role and responsibilities; as an employee, you potentially represent your employer if you name the area of practice, therefore to remain within your employment contract requirements, it is worth outlining in your biography that all views are your own. Remember, this is a public platform and confidentiality must be maintained at all times for both colleagues and patients, so you must consider carefully what you post to remain within NMC (2019b) social media guidance – see annotated reading at the end of the chapter – think about whether anybody could identify an individual from the content you post. If you do wish to use conversations from social media, keep a record or use screenshots to use as evidence for revalidation. If you observe chats but do not participate through posts, this could still count towards your non-participatory CPD if you reflect on what you learnt from the chat. Any background reading you complete to participate in a chat will also count towards non-participatory CPD hours.

Participating in consultations by organisations such as the NMC or RCN can also be used for CPD. Keep a copy of your response as evidence of your participation. Additionally, organisations such as the RCN who have professional forums, participating within their activities can also be used.

Case study: Jamal

Jamal has been registered with the NMC as a Nursing Associate for nearly three years and received notification for revalidation. They have been working within the same area of practice since qualification, however, during this time they have been actively pursuing further learning opportunities. Jamal has an account with X which they use to keep up to date with new publications. They particularly like the Kings Fund as they produce short videos as well as reports that helps process what the policies actually mean in practice. Recently, Jamal joined 'Adapt to thrive in digital health and care – community of interest'. This community meets once a month for 50 minutes to explore how practitioners of all levels can utilise digital health and care resources. Although there is a financial cost involved for Jamal, this has given access to a network of practitioners and managers who have shared ideas and challenges that they have addressed through digital solutions.

Making this commitment was a big undertaking as work is so busy, however, Jamal's line manager has been supportive in giving study time for this each month. In return, Jamal shares what they have learnt from the sessions within the team meeting once a month. During their appraisal, the line manager praises Jamal for taking a proactive approach, so when they ask what aspirations Jamal has for the coming year, Jamal asks if being considered for the BSc pre-registration nursing apprenticeship would be possible. Previously, the line manager had identified they were unable to support any application from Jamal as they lacked experience. On this occasion, the manager states they would have to discuss this with the education team and check with HR as they had not planned to support an apprentice in the coming year; however, Jamal has been forward thinking and that perhaps they may be able to relook at this – if they are unable to do so for the coming intake, they state they will support an application for the following year.

Jamal comes away feeling a little despondent, sure that this is a way of avoiding saying no. They feel they have no real control over what is happening, so they discuss whether there is anything else they can do to support their case with the education team. They suggest becoming a digital champion for the department, sharing new insights further than their immediate team. A couple of months go by without any news; however, one day, the line manager approaches Jamal asking if there was a place available to start with the next intake, would they be interested, even though this is a last minute opportunity; Jamal is all prepared, follows this up and is accepted onto the course to start two months later. They discover that the place only became available due to someone moving out of the area and internally, the education team had suggested Jamal as the most suitable candidate due to the proactive way they have worked over the last 8 months.

Jamal reflects that although they felt they were in the right place at the right time, the opportunity was actually the result of their involvement with the Kings Fund community and their subsequent activity as the digital champion within the department. As a large organisation, this had made Jamal more visible to both their line manager and the education team, where they could have easily been missed if they had not been so proactive.

NMC revalidation

All registrants, whether a nursing associate, nurse or midwife, are required to revalidate their registration every 3 years. The purpose of revalidation is to improve public protection. This is done through making sure that you remain fit to practise throughout your career to demonstrate that you are safe and effective in the care you deliver within your practice and to maintain active registration. This is required to be able to practise within the UK, although nursing associates currently only practise in England. If your registration lapses, even for one day, you cannot practise until you are readmitted to the register, which can take up to 6 weeks. It is a legal requirement that you are NMC registered to work within the UK, this can also occur when your annual registration fee is due, so make sure you remain aware of due dates; the NMC has a number of payment options, including quarterly direct debit, and they email a reminder before each payment is due.

The experiences outlined earlier can all contribute towards your required revalidation CPD hours; however, regardless of how much CPD you have completed, you may feel daunted by your first revalidation experience. It is worth discussing with others who have already completed their revalidation as they will be able to reassure and guide you. If you are feeling anxious, try to think about this as an opportunity to see where you are at, review your longer-term goals and plans and make any adjustments needed to keep you on track with your career aspirations.

When you start preparing for revalidation, starting soon after you qualify – three years can creep up on you – you will need to identify who you are going to ask to review your reflections and activities. Although this can wait until nearer the time, having an idea early can help you to build the relationships needed for you to feel safe and confident in your reflections. This is so you can be open and honest, as well as open to constructive criticism, therefore, this shouldn't be a friend who will simply smile and tick all the right boxes as you will learn nothing from the process.

Activity 8.4   Research

If you have not already researched what is required for NMC revalidation, look at the NMC website (links in annotated reading) to identify what you are required to do. There are also some short videos available that explain the revalidation process if you prefer learning in this way.

This activity is a personal reflection, so there is no outline answer at the end of the chapter.

Revalidation should help reinforce your scope of practice, as well as maintain your fitness to practise. It should also help you to incorporate the NMC (2018a) *The Code* into your daily practice, encourage you to engage with relevant professional networks for discussions that will prevent you feeling isolated professionally; try to look beyond your immediate environment to see what else is happening in other geographical areas – a good website for this is NHS Fabstuff (2024) – see annotated reading. All this activity should help enhance your engagement with the NMC *The Code* and *Standards of Proficiency for Nursing Associates* (2018a, 2024a) but also engage your employer in these standards – you are an advocate for your profession, therefore the stronger application of the standards within your employer organisation, the stronger support and access to CPD can be identified and achieved through appraisals.

Revalidation requirements

Activity 8.4 will have shown you that there are a number of activities that you will have to complete as part of the revalidation process.

1. Practice hours – 450 hours may seem like a lot, but if you are working full time, this will be accumulated quickly; however, remember this is over a three-year period, so it is useful to identify hours in each year. This demonstrates you are consistently working within practice, a key part of retaining skills.
2. 35 hours of CPD – if you break it up, is just over 11 hours per year. When you are working in a busy environment, or short of staff, it can be difficult to identify time for this. Remember, this does not have to be formal learning, it can include a range of activities including team meetings, case conferences, webinars, all of which will aid you in achieving the 20 hours of participatory CPD. Make sure you keep a record with some notes so you can demonstrate these activities.
3. Collecting five pieces of practice-related feedback – like practice hours, these should cover each year to demonstrate continued good practice but also creates a resource for you to reflect on your continued growth and development. It doesn't need to be written feedback, it could be verbal but you will need to record who, when, what it was and how this influenced your ongoing practice. You may occasionally receive negative feedback, which is something you could use for your revalidation as you can demonstrate how you used this to improve your practice. You can also use formal feedback from appraisals, or thank you cards from patients or carers, although ensure these are anonymised.
4. Written reflective accounts will be something as a SNA you are using all the time for your practice assessment documents. Once you are qualified, it may be tempting to step away from regularly writing reflection; however, this is probably the most powerful tool you can use for revalidation. Taking time to reflect regularly, or keeping a reflective journal, will give you a significant resource for your revalidation reflection pieces. It is advisable to complete one each year, this will support your engagement with the process and help with further opportunity to re-reflect on this at the point of revalidation. The templates on the NMC website are useful as these also prompt you to think about how this links to the *Code* (NMC, 2018a). Remember, this does not have to be a negative event, it can be on what you did well, an experience you had where you learnt something you then were able to use in practice, or how you feel you have grown as a professional. It doesn't have to be long or complex but it does need to demonstrate growth and development, so using a reflective model could help you with analysing and looking forward to what else you can achieve.
5. Your reflective discussion on your reflective accounts is a great opportunity to share your learning with a colleague, it does not necessarily need to be your line manager, although that may support continued access to learning opportunities as they are able to see your approach to maintaining and developing yourself and your practice. Whoever you identify, they must be an NMC registrant; this can include another nursing associate. It can be an informal discussion over coffee and an opportunity to strengthen a relationship with a colleague. Remember, you can also be asked by other nursing associates for their reflective discussion – this is another good opportunity for your own development and reflection on what it means for you too! You must also remember to respect confidentiality of those your reflections relate to.
6. When it comes to confirmation that all the requirements for NMC revalidation have been met, your confirmer must review all your documents and evidence. Your reflective discussion person can also be your confirmer. It is important to remember that revalidation is not an assessment of your fitness to practise, it is to support and promote good practice to strengthen confidence in the profession. Your confirmer should be your line manager, although this is not a requirement. It also does not need

to be someone who is an NMC registrant. The NMC has a list of appropriate confirmers; however, it is clear this cannot be a close friend or member of your family due to conflict of interest; something the NMC has included in their guidance.

The role of confirmer is important, and therefore, if you are asked to be a confirmer for a colleague, you need to be aware of the role and responsibilities that go with it. You will need to check that all the requirements have been completed, including reviewing evidence that demonstrates this. This is not an assessment of the person's competence, the quality of their work or their fitness to practise, you just need to see whether they can show they have met the requirements. The process should encourage the process of sharing good practice through reflection, which enables improvement in an individual's practice but could also trigger reflection on your own practice.

Challenges you may face with revalidation

If you do not work in an area that delivers hands-on clinical care, you will still need to revalidate, for example, if you are completing a BSc pre-registration nursing programme. Once you qualify as a registered nurse, you will then need to demonstrate 450 hours for each part of your registration, however, if you are using one role for both your nursing associate and registered nurse role, you need to identify whether it can count for both; see annotated reading for further guidance at the end of the chapter. This may be more difficult if your role is a temporary one, for example you work solely through an agency or bank work. As long as you complete the minimum number of practice hours and CPD hours, you will still be able to complete revalidation.

Mandatory training required for your employment cannot be used as CPD, however, mandatory training that is required for your scope of practice can be. For example, if you work with children and young people, mandatory training on Safeguarding at a higher level than required for standard mandatory training, such as level 3, can be used.

One change you need to be aware of is to take care that you remember your revalidation is due on the first day of the month that your registration expires, for example, if your registration was on the 24th September, your application must be submitted on the 1st of September; however, the NMC does notify you 60 days before your registration is due. You do not need to keep your documents electronically, the NMC templates can be downloaded and printed. You are not required to send any of your portfolio to the NMC as this is a self-declaration online; however, they select a sample each month to review and you can be contacted to provide evidence.

If you retain your records electronically, it is worth saving a copy elsewhere, for example, email a copy to yourself. That way, you can access it even if you accidently delete or lose access to the device where it was saved. Remember that your record includes personal data on your confirmer and reflective partner, therefore you must ensure these are kept securely.

Currently, the NMC is completing a review of revalidation requirements (NMC, 2025). It is important to access the latest revalidation documents from the NMC website at the time you are preparing for revalidation to ensure you are using the latest version.

Concerns of role ambiguity and differentiation

Over the time the nursing associate role has taken to develop and been in place, there have been concerns raised about the scope of the role and how this differs from the registered nurse role. As the nursing associate role evolves and develops in different practice environments, these questions are raised again. For you, it is important to recognise how your role differs as this keeps you safe within the standards. As discussed in Chapter 5, the best way to understand the differences is to look at the *Standards of Proficiency for Nursing Associates* alongside the *Standards of Proficiency for Registered Nurses* (NMC, 2024a, 2024b). If you do this, you will see there are clear boundaries to both roles; however, you are the advocate for ensuring you remain within the scope of your role. If you have an enhanced role, then your employer should be providing specific guidance on the scope of this and support through education and competency assessment. You will be an advocate for the role and how this is developed in the future. Working within your boundaries and extending your knowledge through CPD may enable further competencies to be developed, which may lead to policies within your organisation that extend the scope of the nursing associate role. As the demands on health and care services increase, the knowledge and skills practitioners require to meet those needs will also evolve, which will encompass both the registered nurse and registered nursing associate roles. Proactively managing your CPD will support your ability to move forward with these changes when they occur.

Chapter summary

This chapter has drawn on previous chapters to consider how you can support your career development, actions you need to take and recognise your autonomy as a learner following qualification and registration with the NMC. The role of your locus of control has been explored to identify how you perceive the control you have over your aspirations, overcoming barriers to change to be in charge of your career and how you work towards your aspirations. Using SMART goals to develop a 5-year plan to guide CPD activities that work towards your longer term aims, including incorporating requirements for NMC revalidation. What is involved in revalidation, along with challenges in the scope of the nursing associate role within practice, have been considered within the context of employment and CPD to ensure meeting NMC (2018a, 2024a) *The Code* and *Standards of Proficiency for Nursing Associates* for your continued delivery of safe, effective person-centred care throughout your career.

Activities: Brief outline answers

Activity 8.2 Case study analysis (page 121)

Identify which areas of the case study that show an internal locus of control.

Used a strengths and weakness analysis – identified transferable skills and matched to the best role.

Requested an informal discussion and the potential they have in applying for the post. Used SMART targets to build necessary knowledge and skills to secure an interview.

Identify which areas of the case study show an external locus of control.

Mamoud thought they were lucky to be able to visit the unit.

Activity 8.3 Locus of control quiz (page 123)

Example of a completed locus of control quiz:

Test results showed 86% internal locus of control and 14% external locus of control. Reflecting on these, I feel my attitude has changed over time; In the past, I saw opportunities as being in the right place at the right time; just lucky to get the opportunity. Now I can see that these opportunities were the result of my hard work, I studied and created opportunities to prove my worth to my managers. This resulted in putting myself forward for other opportunities; being proactive resulted in further opportunities for study, funded and supported by my manager.

Annotated reading

Locus of control

There are a number of quizzes available online that enable you to explore your own locus of control. This Locus of control quiz is based on Rotter's inventory and linked to learning, therefore you may find this a useful resource www.idrlabs.com/locus-of-control/test.php

NICE OpenAthens

Your employer should be able to create an OpenAthens account. If they do not, you can still request an account directly, giving details of your employment and role. This will be assessed to see whether you meet the criteria for an account. https://openathens.nice.org.uk/

NMC Revalidation guidance and video

The NMC revalidation pages have links to templates as well as guidance on their requirements www.nmc.org.uk/revalidation/

This YouTube video explains the guidance to support you through the process of revalidation www.nmc.org.uk/revalidation/resources/films/

NHS Fabstuff

NHS Fabstuff was developed to promote all the good practice that occurs within the NHS and other care services. It is a great resource to find information on what innovative practice that solves practice issues, improves safety and compassionate care, as well as supporting staff well-being and patient experience, is out there but also an opportunity for you to share your own innovations from practice, for example through projects or research you complete https://fabnhsstuff.net/

NMC social media guidance

This link is for NMC Social Media Guidance and should be read along with your employer's policy and guidance to ensure you work within the identified boundaries www.nmc.org.uk/standards/guidance/social-media-guidance/

NMC duel registration revalidation guidance

The NMC Guidance on duel registrations revalidation requirements outlines what you need to consider when deciding whether you require different practice hours, and CPD for each www.nmc.org.uk/globalassets/sitedocuments/revalidation/multiple-registratio ns-and-additional-qualifications-guidance.pdf

Practice assessor and supervisor

There are a number of resources available in different geographical areas; contact your education department or your local university for one in your local area. This practice assessor/supervisor online course run in the East of England is just one example www.aru.ac.uk/business-employers/practicehub/nursing-associate/online-practice-supe rvisor-practice-assessor-course

Glossary

Accountability   Having overall responsibility for something and being required to rationalise the actions and/or decisions made.

AEI   (Approved Education Institution) NMC reference to universities and other education providers.

Critical analysis   Constructively question and debate something, examining the positive and negative aspects, to evaluate a topic, subject or event.

Delegation   Requesting someone to carry out a care intervention or activity on your behalf. You are accountable for that care intervention or activity, while the person you have delegated to is responsible for it.

Emotional intelligence   The ability to recognise and understand your own emotions and those of other people.

Evidence-based practice   Clinical or therapeutic practice that is based on the results and findings of systematic, valid and trustworthy research studies or projects.

Identity   A healthcare professional's sense of self, including their beliefs, values and behaviours. This is influenced by their profession's characteristics and norms to shape how they think, act and feel as a professional.

Leadership   The action and ability to guide, inspire and influence others to deliver exceptional care using effective communication and collaboration.

Lifelong learning   NMC registrants continuously to develop their knowledge, skills and competence throughout their careers to maintain their registration and provide safe, effective care.

Locus of control   An individual's perception of how much control they have over events in their lives. This ranges from an internal belief they can influence outcomes to an external belief that external forces are the main causes.

Perspective   A particular way of considering something.

Reflection   A process that helps gain insight into attitudes, behaviours, beliefs, values and actions through analytical thinking.

Reflexivity   The ability to examine your own feelings, reactions and/or motives to understand how these influence your actions and thoughts in a situation.

Research   The systematic investigation into, and study of, materials or sources to establish facts and reach new conclusions or confirm existing conclusions.

Resilience   The capacity of individuals and/or organisations to adapt to challenges and changes.

Responsible   The obligation to complete a care intervention or activity within your scope of practice, under supervision of the person with accountability.

Role model   A person whose behaviour, skills, knowledge and/or actions are admired and emulated by others.

SpLD   An umbrella term for neurological conditions that affect how information is learnt and processed.

Toxic culture   A work environment characterised by negativity, dysfunction and lack of trust. This can manifest in behaviours like bullying, harassment and/or lack of respect which negatively impacts employee well-being and productivity.

Values   The regard that something is held to deserve; the importance or worth.

References

Bandura, A. (1977) 'Self-efficacy: Toward a unifying theory of behavioral change', *Psychological Review*, 84(2), pp.191–215.

Belasen, A. (2021) *Resilience in Healthcare Leadership: Practical Strategies and Self-Assessment Tools for Identifying Strengths and Weaknesses.* Productivity Press.

Benner, P. (1982) 'From novice to expert', *American Journal of Nursing*, 82(3), pp.402–407.

Bloom, B.S. (1956) *Taxonomy of Educational Objectives, Handbook: The Cognitive Domain.* New York: David McKay.

Bodalski, E.A., Flory, K., Canu, W.H., Willcutt, E.G. and Hartung, C.M. (2023) 'ADHD symptoms and procrastination in college students: The roles of emotion dysregulation and self-esteem', *Journal of Psychopathology and Behavioral Assessment*, 45(1), pp.48–57. https://doi.org/10.1007/s10862-022-09996-2

Borton, T. (1970). *Reach, Touch and Teach.* London: Hutchinson.

Bowlby, J. (1988). *A Secure Base: Parent-child Attachment and Healthy Human Development.* New York: Basic Books.

Care Quality Commission (2022a) *Regulation 20: Duty of Candour.* [Online] Available at: www.cqc.org.uk/guidance-providers/all-services/regulation-20-duty-candour

Care Quality Commission (2022b) *Our Purpose and Role.* [Online] Available at: www.cqc.org.uk/about-us/our-purpose-role/who-we-are

Cavendish, C. (2013) *An Independent Review into Healthcare Assistants and Support Workers in the NHS and Social Care Settings.* [Online] Available at: https://assets.publishing.service.gov.uk/media/5a7b9df6e5274a7202e18537/Cavendish_Review.pdf

C2D (2021) *The process of transition.* [Online] Available at: www.c2d.co.uk/techniques/process-of-transition/

Chipps, J., le Roux, L., Agabus, J. and Bimerew. M. (2022) 'Nursing informatics skills relevance and competence for final year nursing students', *Curationis*, 45(1), pp.e1–e8. http://doi.org/10.4102/curationis.v45i1.2277

Christensen, D. (2020) 'If you're trying to be productive, stop multitasking', *ONS Voice*, 35(7), p.28.

Cowls, H., Tobin, S. and Cusack, N. (2023) *Leadership for Nursing Associates.* London: Learning Matters; Sage.

Critical Care Networks (2024) *National Competency Framework for Registered Nursing Associates in Adult Critical Care.* [Online] Available at: www.wyccn.org/uploads/6/5/1/9/65199375/17_nursng_associate_registrant_in_critical_care_competencies_v2_2024_final_updated.pdf

Cuddy, A. (2012) *Fake It Till You Make It.* [Online] Available at: www.youtube.com/watch?v=RVmMeMcGcoY

Cummings, J (2012) *Compassion in practice.* [Online] Available at: www.england.nhs.uk/wp-content/uploads/2012/12/compassion-in-practice.pdf

Darvill, A., Stephens, M. and Leigh, J.A. (2021) *Transition to Nursing Practice: From Student to Registered Nurse.* London: Sage.

Delves-Yates, C. (2022) *Essentials of Nursing Practice*, 3rd edn. London: Sage.

Department of Health and Social Care (2023) *NHS Constitution for England.* [Online] Available at: www.gov.uk/government/publications/the-nhs-constitution-for-england

Doran, G.T. (1981) 'There's a S.M.A.R.T. way to write management's goals and objectives', *Management Review,* 70(11), p.35.

Duckworth, A. (2016) *Grit: The Power of Passion and Perseverance.* Scribner Book Company.

Edwards-Maddox, S. (2023) 'Burnout and impostor phenomenon in nursing and newly licensed registered nurses: A scoping review', *Journal of Clinical Nursing,* 32(5–6), pp.653–665. https://doi.org/10.1111/jocn.16475

Equality Act 2010 [Online] Available at: www.legislation.gov.uk/ukpga/2010/15/contents

Eyler, J.R. (2018). *How Humans Learn: The Science and Stories Behind Effective College Teaching.* West Virginia University Press.

Flaherty, C. and Taylor, M. (Eds) (2024) *Developing Academic Skills for Nursing Associates,* 2nd edn. London: Learning Matters.

Gabriel, K.F. (2017) *Teaching Unprepared Students: Strategies for Promoting Success and Retention in Higher Education.* Bloomfield: Routledge.

Ganguly, S. (2017) 'Understanding nonverbal cues: A key to success in interviews', *IUP Journal of Soft Skills,* 11(2), p.2. ISSN 0973-8479.

Gibbs, G. (1988) *Learning by Doing: A Guide to Teaching and Learning.* Oxford: Oxford Centre for Staff and Learning Development.

Golding, L. (2024) 'Schwartz Rounds: Supporting the emotional wellbeing of our future healthcare workforce', *Future Healthcare Journal,* 11(1), 100010, ISSN 2514-6645, https://doi.org/10.1016/j.fhj.2024.100010

Goleman, D. (2020) 'What people (still) get wrong about emotional intelligence', *Harvard Business Review Digital Articles,* pp.2–4.

González, A.M. (2013). *The Emotions and Cultural Analysis.* London: Routledge.

Grant, A.M. (2011) 'Is it time to REGROW the GROW model? Issues related to teaching coaching session structures', *The Coaching Psychologist,* 7(2), pp.118–126.

Halilović, L. (2021) *Core Values, Your Inner Compass.* [Online] Available at: https://www.ted.com/talks/larisa_halilovic_core_values_your_inner_compass

Harold, A. (2016) 'Nurses on the cheap? The nursing associate role examined', *Nursing Practice.* [Online] Available at: www.nursinginpractice.com/professional/training/nurses-on-the-cheap-the-nursing-associate-role-examined/

Health Education England (2015) *Raising the Bar: Shape of Caring: A review of the Future Education and Training of Registered Nurses and Care Assistants.* [Online] Available at: www.hee.nhs.uk/sites/default/files/documents/2348-Shape-of-caring-review-FINAL.pdf

Hedayioglu, J., Yearsley, S., Nash, G. and Waldock, K. (2023) 'Staff experiences of the nursing associate role in a community setting', *Nursing Standard,* 38(9), pp.28–34. https://doi.org/10.7748/ns.2023.e12090

Johannessen, J.A. (2022), 'What is tacit knowledge?', *The Philosophy of Tacit Knowledge,* pp. 5–27. Emerald Publishing Limited. https://doi.org/10.1108/978-1-80382-677-620221004

King, R., Laker, S., Taylor, B., Ryan, T., Wood, E., Tod, A., Senek, M., Snowden, S. and Robertson, S. (2024) 'Development of the nursing associate professional identity: A longitudinal qualitative study', *Nursing Open,* 11(3), p.e2131. https://doi.org/10.1002/nop2.2131

Kolb, D. A. (1984) *Experiential Learning: Experience as a Source of Learning and Development.* New Jersey: Prentice-Hall.

Kolb, D.A. (2015) *Experiential Learning: Experience as a Source of Learning and Development,* 2nd edn Pearson Education Ltd.

Kübler-Ross, E. and Kessler, D. (2005) *On Grief and Grieving: Finding the Meaning of Grief through the Five Stages of Loss.* New York, NY: Scribner.

Leighton Gamel, A. (2016) *Learning Vital Reading Strategies: A Workbook for Students.* Lanham, Maryland: Rowman & Littlefield Publishers.

Luft, J. and Ingham, H. (1955) 'The Johari window, a graphic model of interpersonal awareness', *Proceedings of the western training laboratory in group development.* Los Angeles: UCLA.

Malpas, M.D. (2017) *Self-fulfilment with Dyslexia: A Blueprint for Success.* Jessica Kingsley Publishers.

Maslach, C. and Leiter, M.P. (2016) 'Understanding the burnout experience: recent research and its implications for psychiatry', *World Psychiatry*, 15(2), pp.103–111.

Mehrabian, A. (1972) *Nonverbal Communication.* Routledge. https://doi.org/10.4324/9781351308724

Mid Staffordshire NHS Foundation Trust Public Inquiry. (2013). *Report of the Mid Staffordshire NHS Foundation Trust Public Inquiry: Executive summary (HC 947).* The Stationery Office. [Online] Available at: https://assets.publishing.service.gov.uk/government/uploads/system/uploads/attachment_data/file/279124/0947.pdf

National Institute for Care Excellence (2024) *Register for a NHS England OpenAthens account.* [Online] Available at: https://openathens.nice.org.uk/

Neal, M. and Gonot-Schoupinsky, F. (2023) 'Laughter and mental health: A case study of Merv Neal', *Mental Health and Social Inclusion*, 27(4), pp.407–416. https://doi.org/10.1108/MHSI-06-2022-0039

Newton, S. and Moore, G. (2010) 'Nursing students' reading and English aptitudes and their relationship to discipline-specific formal writing ability: A descriptive correlational study', *Nursing Education Perspectives*, 31(4), pp.221–225.

NHS (2019) *Long term plan: Chapter 5: Digitally-enabled care will go mainstream across the NHS.* [Online] Available at: www.longtermplan.nhs.uk/online-version/chapter-5-digitally-enabled-care-will-go-mainstream-across-the-nhs/

NHS England (2022a) *Freedom to speak up.* [Online] Available at: www.england.nhs.uk/our-work/freedom-to-speak-up/

NHS England (2022b) *Our NHS people promise.* [Online] Available at: www.england.nhs.uk/our-nhs-people/online-version/lfaop/our-nhs-people-promise/

NHS England (2023) *NHS equality, diversity, and inclusion improvement plan.* [Online] Available at: www.england.nhs.uk/long-read/nhs-equality-diversity-and-inclusion-improvement-plan/

NHS FabStuff (2024) *The academy of fabulous stuff.* [Online] Available at: https://fabnhsstuff.net/

NMC (2018a) *The Code: Standards of professional behaviour for nurses, midwives and nursing associates.* [Online] Available at: www.nmc.org.uk/standards/code/

NMC (2019a) *Enabling professionalism.* [Online] Available at: https://www.nmc.org.uk/globalassets/sitedocuments/other-publications/enabling-professionalism.pdf

NMC (2019b) *Read Social media guidance online.* [Online] Available at: www.nmc.org.uk/standards/guidance/social-media-guidance/read-social-media-guidance-online/

NMC (2019c) *Guidance on the professional duty of candour.* [Online] Available at: www.nmc.org.uk/standards/guidance/the-professional-duty-of-candour/

NMC (2019d) *Regulators unite to support reflective practice across health and care.* [Online] Available at: www.nmc.org.uk/news/press-releases/joint-statement-reflective-practice/

NMC (2021) *Ensuring your decisions to refer are fair and unbiased.* [Online] Available at: www.nmc.org.uk/employer-resource/deciding-to-refer/fair-unbiased-decisions/

NMC (2024a) *Standards of proficiency for nursing associates.* [Online] Available at: www.nmc.org.uk/standards/standards-for-nursing-associates/standards-of-proficiency-for-nursing-associates/

NMC (2024b) *Standards of proficiency for registered nurses.* [Online] Available at: www.nmc.org.uk/standards/standards-for-nurses/standards-of-proficiency-for-registered-nurses/

NMC (2024c) *Standards of student supervision and assessment.* [Online] Available at: https://www.nmc.org.uk/standards-for-education-and-training/standards-for-student-supervision-and-assessment/

NMC (2025) *Future standards* [Online] Available at: https://www.nmc.org.uk/standards/future-standards/#:~:text=Code%20and%20revalidation%20review,revalidation%20process%20in%20October%202027

Nursing and Midwifery Order (2001) [Online] Available at: https://www.legislation.gov.uk/uksi/2002/253/contents

RCN (2025) *Interviews*. [Online] Available at: https://startingout.rcn.org.uk/Your-Career/Interviews [Resource only available to logged in members].

Richardson, C., Wicking, K., Biedermann, N., and Langtree, T. (2023) 'Coaching in nursing: an integrative literature review', *Nursing Open*, 10(10), pp.6635–6649. https://doi.org/10.1002/nop2.1925

Rolfe, G., Jasper, M. and Freshwater, D. (2011) *Critical Reflection in Practice: Generating Knowledge for Care*, 2nd edn. Basingstoke: Palgrave Macmillan.

Rotter, J.B. (1966). 'Generalized expectancies for internal versus external control of reinforcement', *Psychological Monographs: General and Applied*, 80 (1), p. 1.

Schön, D.A. (1983) *The Reflective Practitioner: How Professionals Think in Action*. London: Temple Smith.

Schön, D.A. (1987). *Educating the Reflective Practitioner: Toward a New Design for Teaching and Learning in the Professions*. London: Jossey-Bass.

Schweizer, S., Lawson, R.P. and Blakemore, S.-J. (2023) 'Uncertainty as a driver of the youth mental health crisis', *Current Opinion in Psychology*, 53. https://doi.org/10.1016/j.copsyc.2023.101657

Sheehy-Skeffington and Rea (2017) *How Poverty Affects People's Decision-Making Processes*. [Online] Available at: www.jrf.org.uk/savings-debt-and-assets/how-poverty-affects-peoples-decision-making-processes

Southwick, S.M., Sippel, L., Krystal, J., Charney, D., Mayes, L. and Pietrzak, R. (2016) 'Why are some individuals more resilient than others: The role of social support', *World Psychiatry*, 15(1), pp.77–79.

Stolovitch, H.D. and Keeps, E.J. (2021) *Know-How. Association for Talent Development*. USA: ATD Press.

Topping, A. (2023) Exploring the implementation of the nursing associate role in general practice, *Primary Health Care*. [Online] Available at: https://journals.rcni.com/primary-health-care/evidence-and-practice/exploring-the-implementation-of-the-nursing-associate-role-in-general-practice-phc.2023.e1817/full

Turner, S.B., and Kaylor, S.D. (2015) 'Neuman systems model as a conceptual framework for nurse resilience', *Nursing Science Quarterly*, 28(3), pp.213–217. https://doi.org/10.1177/0894318415585620

van Gennep. A. (2019) *Rites of Passage,* 2nd edn Chicago, IL: University of Chicago Press. (Translated 1960 & 1988 by Vizedom, M.B. and Caffee, G.L.).

Whitmore, J., Kauffman, C. and David, S.A. (2013) 'GROW grows up: from winning the game to pursuing transpersonal goals'. In: S.A. David, D. Clutterbuck and D. Megginson (eds), *Beyond Goals: Effective Strategies for Coaching and Mentoring*. Farnham: Gower Publishing Limited. https://doi.org/10.4324/9781315569208

Bibliography

Alexander, V. (2018) *How to outsmart your own unconscious bias*. [Online] Available at: www.youtube.com/watch?v=GP-cqFLS8Q4

Benner, P. (1984) *From Novice to Expert: Excellence and Power in Clinical Nursing Practice*. Addison-Wesley Publishing Company.

Blakemore, S. and Choudhury, S. (2006) 'Development of the adolescent brain: Implications for executive function and social cognition', *Journal of Child Psychology and Psychiatry*, 47(3–4), pp.296–312. https://doi.org/10.1111/j.1469-7610.2006.01611.x

Dean, E. (2023) 'Why is imposter syndrome so common among nurses?: Imposter feelings can erode self-confidence and increase likelihood of burnout, but there are ways of defusing it', *Cancer Nursing Practice*, 22(6), pp.16–17. https://doi.org/10.7748/cnp.22.6.16.s7

Howatson-Jones, L. (2016) *Reflective Practice in Nursing*, 3rd edn. London: Sage/Learning Matters.

Iheakanwa, J.U., Obro, S. and Akpochafo, W.P. (2021) 'Reading ability, study habits and students' academic performance in social studies', *Library Philosophy and Practice*, 2021, pp.1–21.

Johns, C. (1995) 'Framing learning through reflection within Carper's fundamental ways of knowing in nursing', *Journal of Advanced Nursing*, 22 (2), pp.226–234.

Mahon, P. and O'Neill, M. (2020) 'Through the looking glass: the rabbit hole of reflective practice', *British Journal of Nursing*, 29(13), pp.777–783. https://doi.org/10.12968/bjon.2020.29.13.777

McCabe, M.P. and O'Connor, E.J. (2012) 'Why are some people with neurological illness more resilient than others?', *Psychology Health & Medicine*, 17(1), pp.17–34.

McKinnon, J. (2016) *Reflection for Nursing Life: Principles, Process and Practice*. London: Routledge.

Mittelmark, M.B. and Bauer, G.F. (2016) 'The meanings of salutogenesis'. In: M.B. Mittelmark, S. Sagy, M. Eriksson, et al. (eds), *The Handbook of Salutogenesis [Internet]*. Cham: Springer; 2017. Chapter 2. Available at: www.ncbi.nlm.nih.gov/books/NBK435854/, https://doi.org/10.1007/978-3-319-04600-6_2

National Academies Press (2018) *How people learn II: learners, contexts, and cultures* (A consensus study report of the National Academies of Sciences, Engineering, Medicine). [Online] Available at: https://nap.nationalacademies.org/read/24783/chapter/1

Peate, I. (2019) *Learning to Care: The Nursing Associate*. London: Elsevier.

Plutchik, R. (1980) 'A general psychoevolutionary theory of emotion'. In: R. Plutchik and H. Kellerman (eds) *Theories of Emotion*. London: Elsevier, pp.3–33. www.theschwartzcenter.org/about/who-we-are/

Redwood, T., Ward, A., Ali, T., O'Dell, C., Poole, C. and Rebaudo, D. (2024) 'Continued professional development (CPD) provision for nurses: A qualitative exploration', *Heliyon*, 10(12), e32582, ISSN 2405-8440, https://doi.org/10.1016/j.heliyon.2024.e32582

Williams, L., Arribas-Ayllon, M., Artemiou, A. and Spasić, I. (2019) 'Comparing the utility of different classification schemes for emotive language analysis', *Journal of Classification*, 36(3), pp.619–648. https://doi.org/10.1007/s00357-019-9307-0

World Health Organization (2025) *Our values*. [Online] Available at: https://www.who.int/about/values

Index

Index

U

Unconscious bias, 30–34
Underpinning resilience, 39
    biological, personality and sociocultural
        connections, 39

V

Values, 20, 41, 51
    assessment of, 50–54
    commitment to quality of care, 53
    compassion, 53
    everyone counts, 53–54
    improving lives, 53
    NHS constitution, 52–54
    respect and dignity, 52
    working together for patients, 52

van Gennep. A., 89–90
Verbal feedback, 25

W

Weaknesses, 1, 7, 11
Well-being, 38
Western middle-class people, 120
Workload management, 5
Workshops, 124
World Health Organization (WHO),
    53–54
Writing, 6
Written
    communication, 111
    feedback, 25
    reflective accounts, 128

www.ingramcontent.com/pod-product-compliance
Lightning Source LLC
Chambersburg PA
CBHW051755200326
41597CB00025B/4561